EMERGENCY FIRST AID MANUAL

CLB 4064
This edition published 1995 by
Colour Library Books
© 1995 Colour Library Books Ltd,
Godalming, Surrey
All rights reserved
Printed and bound in Singapore
ISBN 1-85833-487-X

Editorial
Steve Parker

Design
Patrick Nugent

Contributing Editor
Philip de Ste Croix

Illustration
Kevin Jones Associates

The publishers would like to thank:
Bob Pearcey and Alan Line for
paramedic advice, supplying
equipment and demonstrating
techniques; Bill O'Neill for wound
make-up and injury simulation; the
Heathrow Training Centre of the
London Ambulance Service for use
of photographic studio and
facilities; Neil Sutherland for taking
the reference photographs for the
illustrations in this book; and those
who helped to model and simulate
the accidents and emergencies:
Stuart Davidson, Sarah de Ste
Croix, Robert Green, Catherine
Line, Matthew Line, Jonathan
Pearcey, and Farzahn Tachakra.

IMPORTANT NOTE TO ALL READERS AND FIRST-AIDERS
First aid is vital, but variable. Each situation is different and must
be assessed on its unique conditions. Books can show basic
techniques and give general guidelines. But these may not be
applicable in some cases. All readers are urged to undertake
approved practical training courses, gain experience and achieve
recognized qualifications. Neither author nor publishers can take
any responsibility for any results, effects or outcomes connected
with any advice or method in this book, howsoever caused.

EMERGENCY FIRST AID MANUAL

Mr. Sapal Tachakra

Fellow of the Royal College of Surgeons
Clinical Director, Accident and Emergency
Department, Central Middlesex Hospital, London

CLB

Colour Library Books

CONTENTS

HOW TO USE THIS BOOK

1 Scan through the main CONTENTS list on the previous pages, to locate the particular emergency or situation.

2 Refer to the INDEX on pages 158-159, at the end of the book, for a detailed alphabetical list of topics.

3 If you are unsure of the problem — for example, you find someone unconscious — turn to pages 16-17.

4 In the case of a multiple emergency, when several casualties may require attention, see pages 10-11 and 14-15.

Almost anyone, anywhere, at any time, can be affected by an emergency. It may be a sudden illness, an accident involving machinery or vehicles, a fire or flood, or even a violent attack. It may affect an adult, an older person, a child, or a baby. When the situation is serious, seconds count.

In an ideal world, all adults should attend a first aid course, for practical instruction and to gain experience. However, this is often a low priority. So when the need arises, we require fast and convenient access to advice which is clearly displayed, highly visual, authoritative, and accurate in most situations. This book is for people who have not had an opportunity to undertake a first aid course, but who would like the reassurance of knowing, in everyday terms, how to deal with medical emergencies.

❶ The numbered stages, in this format, tell you what to do in step-by-step fashion.

❷ The information is clear and concise, to save time.

1 The numbered stages are keyed into short captions, in this format, that accompany the pictures.

2 Each caption and picture describe the stage in more detail, explaining and illustrating what to do.

The *EMERGENCY FIRST AID MANUAL* aims to help you tackle not only life-threatening major emergencies, but also dozens of minor problems and routine first-aid situations — around the home, at work and play, and on the road. The information is portrayed in stage-by-stage format. It explains the vital steps that the sensible first-aider can take to assist a casualty, avoid injury and suffering, and possibly save a life.

But all first-aiders must still be aware of priorities, alternatives, and limitations. Should you call for expert assistance and wait for it to arrive, or would it be better to transport a casualty yourself? Should you try to give on-the-spot treatment, or might this cause problems later? The *EMERGENCY FIRST AID MANUAL* helps to answer these questions and points you, armed with your common sense, in the right direction.

PRINCIPLES OF FIRST AID

REMEMBER THE "3 Ps"

- **PRESERVE LIFE**

- **PREVENT THE CASUALTY'S CONDITION FROM WORSENING**

- **PROMOTE RECOVERY**

PART ONE

GENERAL TECHNIQUES

DEALING WITH EMERGENCIES

Emergencies vary from the extremely minor, such as a cut finger or bruised toe, to a major incident like a road traffic accident, with a number of casualties suffering from various life-threatening conditions. But there are certain basic guidelines that apply to almost any first-aid situation, and these are described opposite.

At all times, try to think rationally, stay calm, and act sensibly. People who panic, or who shout and rush about unnecessarily, offer no help to the casualty. Indeed, they may make matters worse.

THE POSSIBILITY OF INFECTION — ARE YOU AT RISK?

If you are involved in first aid, especially where blood and body fluids are concerned, might you be in danger of contracting or passing on a serious infection such as hepatitis or HIV?

In general, the risks are very, very small. In all cases, you must weigh any possible risks and dangers against the natural urge to help, and possibly save a life.

In most regions, conditions such as HIV are rare among the general population. You may well know the casualty and his or her lifestyle, and so you will be able to assess the risks. In the case of strangers or in foreign places, the situation may be less clear.

Professional medical and paramedical staff are trained in the use of masks, gloves, and similar equipment, to minimize the risks. If these items are available, they should always be used, according to standard guidelines. Take advice from qualified personnel.

1 Assess the overall situation. How many casualties are there? Whose condition is most serious? The casualty who makes most noise may well be in least need of attention, compared to the quiet or unconscious person. Might there be overriding risks such as the danger of fire or explosion?

2 Make a provisional diagnosis. This means you try to identify the condition or disease from which the casualty is suffering. Sometimes it is fairly obvious, such as a head wound. At other times it may be less clear, such as fainting, or finding someone unconscious (see page 16).

3 At the earliest opportunity, arrange to get help or summon expert assistance, as appropriate. Usually, the fastest method is to telephone the emergency services. Make use of bystanders as necessary. If there is no one to hand, you may have to carry out vital life-saving treatment first, before getting help.

4 Give appropriate attention and treatment, with the time and resources available. This may vary from simply staying with and comforting the casualty, to stemming severe bleeding. Be aware that a casualty may have more than one injury or condition, so deal with the most serious ones first.

SAFETY-FIRST FIRST AID

Any type of first aid should take into account the risks and dangers of the situation. Include these in your initial assessment, and act to minimize them as necessary. Take care to avoid becoming another casualty yourself.

Road accidents

Make sure that passing vehicles do not present any danger. Instruct someone to control the traffic. Park your vehicle in such a way as to protect the casualty from traffic. Switch on flashing hazard lights. Locate warning triangles and position these to forewarn approaching vehicles. In darkness, wave a torch to and fro.

Electricity

If you touch a person who is suffering electric shock, you will also experience the shock. So switch off the electricity. Or take precautions against shock by using a non-conducting object (wood, plastic, thick textile) to remove the casualty from the electricity. See page 126.

Fire and collapsing structures

If the casualty is in imminent danger, move him or her to safety. Ensure someone has contacted the fire service. Look and listen for creaks, cracks, and other signs that a building or other structure may collapse. See page 120.

Gas and poisonous fumes

If possible, turn off the gas at its source, or close its ducts and outlets. Move the casualty to fresh air, or open doors and windows to disperse the gas or fumes (but be careful not to fan flames). See pages 51, 52.

Water emergencies

If someone is in difficulty, especially in a fast-flowing river, or among large waves, or in a tidal area, look for aids such as lifebelts or ropes. Beware of swift currents. Be very sure of your own abilities should you decide to attempt a rescue, and get back-up help before you do so. See page 50.

All present and accounted for?

In some emergencies, such as a road crash, casualties may be thrown some distance from a vehicle, or try to crawl clear themselves. Ask others if all the people involved are accounted for.

PRIORITIES FOR THE CASUALTY

The human body has several vital needs, and without them, its life is at risk. The needs centre around the body's continuing requirement for a supply of oxygen, to fuel its vital functions. Oxygen makes up one-fifth of air. It is breathed in through the nose and mouth, and down the throat and windpipe to the lungs, where it passes into the blood there, and then circulates in the bloodstream to all parts of the body, pumped by the heart.

After a few minutes without oxygen, the body's organs and tissues begin to suffer. They start to deteriorate, and much of the damage can be irreversible. The brain, in particular, is very sensitive to lack of oxygen.

In a first aid situation, the immediate priorities concern maintaining the supply of oxygen for the casualty, and ensuring its circulation via the blood. The three main requirements can be summarized as the ABC of first aid, described opposite. These transfer to the ABC memory-aid for resuscitation. Check the Airway first, then Breathing, and then attend to Circulation.

There are two further priorities. If the casualty is bleeding profusely, then the blood loss may endanger life. So the fourth action is to check for and control severe bleeding. Fifth, if the casualty is unconscious but breathing, he or she should be placed in the stable side position (recovery or coma position). This reduces the risk of the airway becoming blocked by vomit or fluids.

A is for Airway. This is the passageway for fresh air in through the nose or mouth, down through the throat, into the windpipe (trachea), and then to the lungs. See page 28.

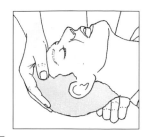

B is for Breathing. This is the muscle-powered chest movement that sucks fresh air through the airway into the lungs, and then expels stale air from them. See page 30.

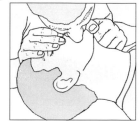

C is for Circulation. This is the flow of blood through the blood vessels (arteries and veins) of the body, powered by the pumping of the heart. See page 32.

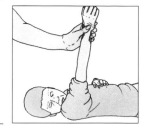

D Control severe bleeding. See page 44.

E Place the casualty in a safe and stable position. See page 40.

IDENTIFYING THE PROBLEM

In many cases where first aid is required, it is relatively simple to identify the problem. In other cases, it may be more difficult to make a diagnosis. You may not be present when the incident occurs, or someone may collapse or suffer pain for no apparent reason.

The skilled first-aider works rapidly but methodically through four main stages. The first three are the history of the incident, the symptoms described by the casualty (if conscious), and the signs noticed by the first-aider. Coupled with the fourth stage, examination of the casualty, these should give you a reasonable idea of the problem. If in doubt, assume the worst and treat accordingly. For an unconscious casualty, see page 62.

HISTORY
"Can you tell me what happened?". This is the sequence of events and the story of what took place. Ask the casualty directly, if he or she is conscious and able to respond. Try not to hurry or panic the casualty. Also ask any bystanders or observers for extra information. Consider the possibility of existing medical conditions such as diabetes, epilepsy, asthma, or angina (heart pain). Look for on-the-spot evidence such as chemical containers, pill bottles, or bloodstains.

SYMPTOMS
"Where does it hurt?" Symptoms are the feelings and sensations experienced by the casualty. They include pain, numbness, paralysis, loss of feeling, giddiness, feeling sick (nausea), and trembling or shaking. Try to remember them, and pass on the information when expert help arrives. If the casualty is unconscious or unable to describe the symptoms fully, you will have to rely more on the signs, which you ascertain yourself.

LEVELS OF RESPONSIVENESS

1 The casualty listens and talks normally and responds well to questions and requests.

2 The casualty responds only to direct questions, and may seem dazed or vague.

3 The casualty seems detached or confused, and may have trouble understanding and answering questions.

4 The casualty can hear and obey direct commands, but is unable to talk or explain the problem.

5 The casualty appears very drowsy or sleepy, and responds only to pain, such as being pinched.

6 The casualty does not respond at all — he or she is unconscious. See page 62.

SIGNS
"What do I notice?" Signs are features of the casualty's condition that are gathered by the first-aider. Use your main senses — look, listen, smell, and feel. Assess the casualty's level of responsiveness, as detailed above. Check the casualty's breathing and pulse. Is there severe bleeding or fluid loss? Is any part of the body swollen or deformed, compared to the same part on the other side? Some signs may be obvious, but others are noticed only by a prompt yet careful examination.

EXAMINATION
"What can I detect?" Quickly carry out a general examination, starting with the head, down the body to the legs and feet. Begin with breathing, ensuring that the airway is clear, and pulse. Examine the eyes, nose, and ears for injury, bleeding, or fluid loss. Is the face flushed, or pale, or bluish? Gently look at and feel the neck, chest, arms, abdomen, and legs for obvious injury, swelling, or deformity. There may be a necklace or bracelet informing of a medical condition (see pages 59, 146).

HANDLING AND MOVING A CASUALTY

For minor injuries, it may be possible to transport the casualty by car to a hospital, medical centre, or similar facility.

In a serious emergency, the general aim of first aid is to preserve life and stabilize the casualty's condition. Assuming that expert assistance is on its way, it is usually best to manhandle or move a casualty as little as possible. Make him or her comfortable, monitor the condition, and wait for the medical team to arrive. The ambulance crew, paramedics, or medical staff have the training and equipment to move and transport a casualty with the minimum of risk.

If you really must move a casualty, follow the basic guidelines described opposite. Remember that the human body is heavy, and an unconscious casualty seems twice the weight.

WARNING
If there is a risk of serious injury, especially to the neck or back, DO NOT move or transport a casualty UNLESS there is an immediate threat to life, such as fire, smoke, fumes, or a collapsing structure (see pages 94, 96).

Moving a casualty who has a serious injury may worsen the condition. Movement or change of position can cause further damage, for example, by widening a wound, encouraging blood loss, or damaging nerves.

GET ORGANIZED

Arrange for as many people as possible to help. Designate the most experienced as leader, who gives instructions and words of command for each stage, so that movements are smooth and coordinated among the team.

OFFER SUPPORT

Make sure that the casualty's injured part is immobilized and supported, so that it is moved as little as possible. Explain what you are doing at each stage, so both the casualty and the team can be prepared and help as necessary.

USE RESOURCES

There are various methods of lifting and carrying a casualty, such as the firefighter's lift, hand-seat, and cradle-carry. If there is no stretcher available, you might be able to improvize one using a chair, door, coats, blankets, wooden poles, and other items. Make sure your equipment and method can take the full weight of the casualty, by carefully testing it first, to avoid further injury should it give way or break.

THE FIRST AID KIT

Several types of first aid kit are available commercially, for use in the home or workplace, or while travelling. If you are assembling your own kit, the items shown here are useful for many situations. In factories, chemical works, engineering shops, and similar places, health and safety regulations usually apply, and more specialized first aid equipment should be available.

The first aid kit should be in a dust-proof, clearly marked container. It should be kept in a clean, dry, well known, and easily accessible place. As items are used, such as sticking plasters, these should be replaced. Every year or two, the whole kit should be checked, and its contents renewed as necessary.

A TYPICAL KIT CONTAINS

Sterile fabric dressings

Sterile eye pad with bandage

Sterile wash/irrigation (sodium chlorite)

Selection of roller bandages

Triangular bandages

Safety pins

Tweezers

Scissors

Sterile plain dressings

Gauze dressings

Burns dressings

Assorted sticking plasters

Dish

Antiseptic lotion and cream

Antihistamine cream

Cotton wool

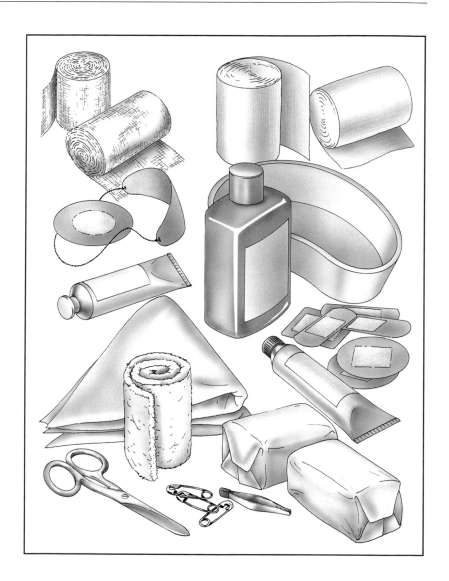

PREVENTING ACCIDENTS

Even in the most well-regulated place, with the most safety-conscious people, accidents can happen. But the chances of an accident, and the need for first aid, can be vastly reduced by following these simple guidelines and precautions. Young and old people are most at risk, so pay special attention to the places where they spend time and move about. *continued* ▶

IN THE HOME

GENERAL

1 Avoid trailing electrical wires and flexes.

2 Fix loose mats, carpet corners, warped tiles, and other floor coverings.

3 Make sure steps, stairs, stairwells, corridors, and similar places are well lit, with secure handrails.

4 Cover unused electrical sockets or use blank plugs.

5 Keep alcohol, glassware, and similar items in a secure place.

6 Ensure that glass doors and glass partitions are visible.

KITCHEN

1 Avoid trailing electrical wires and flexes.

2 Turn saucepan handles so they do not overhang.

3 Use a hob guard.

4 Do not place kettles, pans, and other containers near the edge of the oven top, hob, or work surface.

5 Keep all kitchen and household chemicals in securely fastened, child-proof cupboards.

6 Provide a suitable fire extinguisher or fire blanket.

BATHROOM

1 Keep medicines, pills, and similar substances in a secure, child-proof place (see page 20).

2 Use non-slip mats, handles, and rails for safety in the shower cubicle or bathtub.

3 Do not fill a bathtub with scalding hot water first, and do not leave taps running unattended.

4 Do not bring mains electrical equipment into the bathroom.

5 Beware that foot-mats do not slip on a smooth floor covering.

Preventing accidents continued

GARAGE AND GARDEN

1 Re-label containers clearly if they have new contents. Do not re-use soft drink or similar tempting containers.

2 Ensure paints, fuels, cleaners, and other harmful substances are on safe, high shelves.

3 Provide approved circuit breakers or similar equipment, especially for workshop and garden tools on extension leads.

4 Do not leave rakes, ropes, shears, or other items lying around.

5 Prevent temptation by removing keys or starters from cars, mowers, and similar equipment.

IN THE CAR

1 Use child-proof locks and similar aids.

2 Fit approved child seats or booster seats according to the vehicle's safety guidelines.

3 Ensure all occupants wear seatbelts.

4 Check before opening doors at the roadside, especially on the offside. Move across to use the nearside door in busy traffic.

5 Always check in front and behind before moving off, for bicycles, toys, and even small children playing hide-and-seek.

OUT AND ABOUT

1 Ensure that children are trained in road safety appropriate for their age.

2 Discourage the misuse of playground equipment.

3 Do not eat or handle unknown or suspicious items such as berries or "sweets".

4 Beware of dogs and other animals, even if they seem friendly.

5 Teach children how to respond if they are approached by strangers, or offered sweets or rides.

6 When venturing into remote places, be well prepared, and tell someone of your proposed route and when you expect to return.

ON HOLIDAY

1 Be very cautious about sunbathing. Follow the advice on page 134.

2 Wear beach shoes rather than going barefoot.

3 Do not touch or poke animals, especially fish, urchins, and jellyfish. They can sting or poison, even when dead.

4 When taking part in sports and activities, wear suitable equipment and follow guidelines.

5 Be prepared with sunscreen cream, insect repellents, digestive medicines, and similar substances.

PART TWO

MAJOR EMERGENCIES

PRINCIPLES OF RESUSCITATION

When you encounter a casualty, especially someone who is unconscious, the first priorities are to check the vital signs — breathing and heartbeat.

If the airway to the lungs is not clear, or if there are no breathing movements, or if the heart is not beating, then the vital oxygen which is needed by all body parts to stay alive, will not be circulating around the body. This can result in death within minutes.

The techniques of mouth-to-mouth ventilation and cardiopulmonary (heart-lung) resuscitation aim to replace these vital functions until the casualty begins to breathe and regain heartbeat, or until expert help arrives.

The priorities and necessary actions are termed the ABC of first aid (see page 15), and are described opposite.

The following pages show the principles of resuscitation. (See Contents, Index for page numbers). In summary, priorities are:

1 Quickly check the casualty's airway, breathing, and pulse. Take action as follows:

2 Airway. Sweep your finger around to locate and remove any blockage. Check for possible choking, strangulation, or suffocation.

3 Breathing. If all signs of breathing are absent, carry out mouth-to-mouth ventilation. If the pulse is also absent, alternate mouth-to-mouth ventilation with re-starting the heart, or carry out one while a helper does the other.

4 Circulation. If all signs of pulse are absent, try to keep the blood flowing by heart massage and re-starting the heart. If breathing is also absent, alternate mouth-to-mouth ventilation with re-starting the heart, or carry out one while a helper does the other.

● At all times: Stay calm, get expert advice quickly, and obtain emergency help as soon as possible.

MOUTH-TO-MOUTH VENTILATION

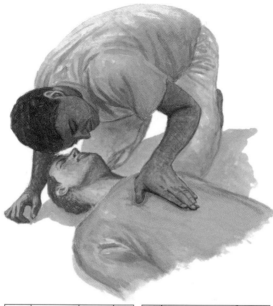

There is enough oxygen in your exhaled breath to supply a casualty's needs for a limited time. Carry out mouth-to-mouth ventilation only if breathing signs are absent (see page 28).

1 Place your hand on the casualty's chest to feel for breathing movements. Put your face close to the mouth to hear and feel any breath. Continue only if breathing has stopped.

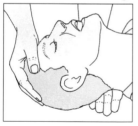

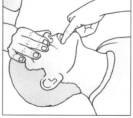

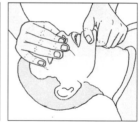

2 Place one hand under the casualty's neck and the other on the forehead. Gently tip the head back to ensure the airways to the lungs are straight and open.

3 Look into the mouth and down the throat for food, dentures, other blockages or chemicals (see page 142). Sweep your finger around to remove any blockages.

4 Move your hand from the forehead to the nose and squeeze it closed. Place your other hand on the chin and lower it to hold the mouth open.

① Check to see if the casualty is breathing.

② If not, tip the head back to open the airway.

③ Clear the casualty's mouth of obstructions and check for other problems (see page 16).

④ Hold the nose closed and mouth open.

⑤ Make an airtight mouth-to-mouth seal.

⑥ Exhale your breath into the casualty's lungs, and ensure this makes the chest rise.

⑦ Carry out five breaths, check for breathing, and continue as described on page 29.

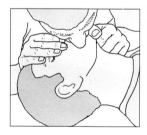 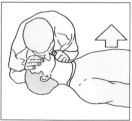 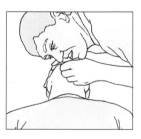

5 Place your mouth over the casualty's mouth to make a good airtight seal. Consider using an artificial (plastic) mask or airway if one is available.

6 Breathe out so your breath enters the casualty's lungs, and look to see if the chest rises. If not, improve the mouth-to-mouth seal and try again.

7 Allow the air to leave. Repeat steps 4-7 four times. Check again for signs of breathing. If absent, carry out another 5 breaths (see page 29).

RESUSCITATING AN ADULT

Like most major first aid techniques, heart massage (external heart compression) is best learned during practical demonstration by qualified instructors. Pressure on the breastbone helps to massage blood around the arteries and veins of the circulation, and may also stimulate the heart to re-start. This technique should not be used if the casualty is conscious or if there are any signs of breathing, heartbeat, or pulse. (See Principles of resuscitation, page 28. For children and babies see pages 36, 38.)

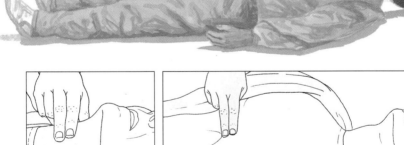

1 Check the carotid pulse. From the projection of the larynx (adam's apple), slide two fingers sideways into the neck's hollow and feel for pulsations.

2 Check the radial pulse also, in the wrist below the mound of the thumb. If there are no signs of pulse, prepare for heart massage. Feel for the lowest end of the breastbone, at the slight projection due to the underlying knob of cartilage. Measure two fingers' width from this, up the chest.

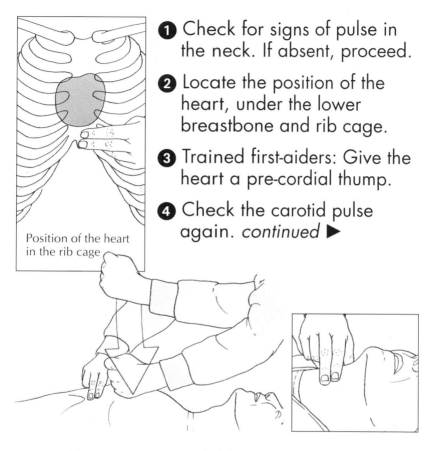

Position of the heart in the rib cage

1 Check for signs of pulse in the neck. If absent, proceed.

2 Locate the position of the heart, under the lower breastbone and rib cage.

3 Trained first-aiders: Give the heart a pre-cordial thump.

4 Check the carotid pulse again. *continued* ▶

3 Trained first-aiders: From a height of about 20 centimetres, bring down your other fist sharply onto the breastbone just above your two fingers. This is a pre-cordial thump. Its physical pressure may stimulate the heart into beating again. Do not use too much pressure and do not repeat this manoeuvre.

4 Check the pulse at the carotid artery in the neck. If there are no signs of pulse, continue with step 5. If a pulse is present, monitor it every few seconds.

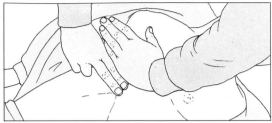
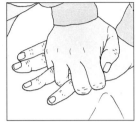

5 If there is no pulse, kneel astride the casualty's head. Repeat step 2 to position two fingers on the lower end of the breastbone. Place the heel (base of the palm) of your other hand next to them, on the upper (head) side.

6 Remove your two fingers. Interlock the fingers of this hand onto those of the hand on the breastbone.

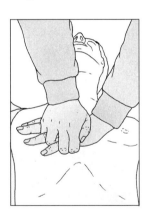
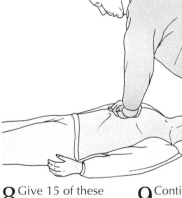

7 With your arms locked straight, rock forward your body weight to push down with the heel of your hand, compressing the chest 5-6 centimetres.

8 Give 15 of these compressions at a rate of 80 per minute. Give 2 inflations (breaths) of mouth-to-mouth ventilation (see page 30).

9 Continue to alternate 15 compressions with 2 inflations. Check the pulse after each minute, and stop if the pulse re-starts.

5 If there is no pulse, place the heel of one hand on the lower breastbone above the heart.

6 Lock the fingers of the other hand onto it.

7 Press down with the heel of your hand to depress the breastbone and compress the chest 5-6 centimetres, to massage blood flow.

8 Give 15 compressions at the rate of 80 per minute, followed by 2 inflations of mouth-to-mouth ventilation. Repeat these alternately, checking the pulse every minute. Stop if the pulse returns, and put the casualty into the stable side position (see page 40).

9 Continue resuscitation until medical help arrives, or you are exhausted, or a doctor advises that there is no hope of recovery.

RESUSCITATION WITH A HELPER
If there are two first aiders, one can carry out the inflations (breaths) of artificial ventilation, while the other performs heart massage (external cardiac compression) to re-start the heart. For an adult, the recommended procedure is one inflation, five compressions, and so on. Check the carotid pulse every minute, and stop if the pulse re-starts.

RESUSCITATING A CHILD

For a child (about 1 to 14 years), modify the adult resuscitation method as follows. See also Principles of resuscitation, page 28.

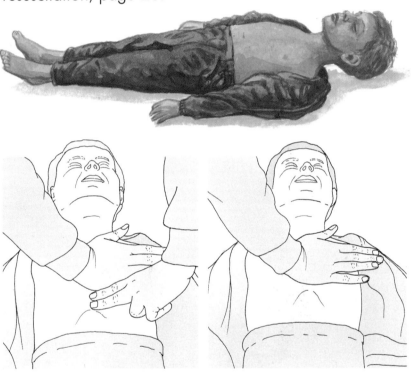

1 Do not carry out resuscitation if the child is conscious, or if there are signs of breathing or a carotid pulse (see page 32). Check the airway and tip the head back. Position your two fingers on the lower breastbone (see page 32).

2 Kneeling beside the child, place the heel of your other hand on the breastbone next to your fingers. Press down with this hand only, about 3-4 centimetres. This is one compression.

1 Check that the child is unconscious, and that breathing and pulse are absent.

2 Place your hand on the lower breastbone.

3 Give 15 compressions of 3-4 centimetres each, at the rate of 100 per minute,

4 Alternate compressions with 2 mouth-to-mouth inhalations. Stop when the pulse returns.

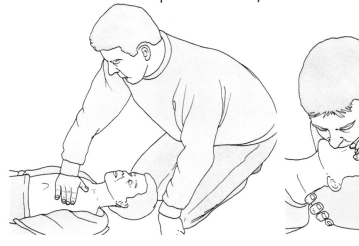

3 Give 15 of these compressions rapidly, at the rate of about 100 per minute. Follow these with 2 inhalations (breaths) of mouth-to-mouth ventilation. Continue to alternate 15 compressions and 2 inhalations. Check the carotid pulse after each minute. If it is present, stop resuscitation.

4 If the pulse is absent, continue with alternating 15 compressions and 2 inhalations, as described in step 9 on page 35.

RESUSCITATING A BABY

For a baby (up to about 1 year), modify the adult resuscitation method (see page 32) as follows. Use the pressure of two fingers only, give inhalations through the baby's nose <u>and</u> mouth, and keep the baby warm to prevent hypothermia. See also Principles of resuscitation, page 28.

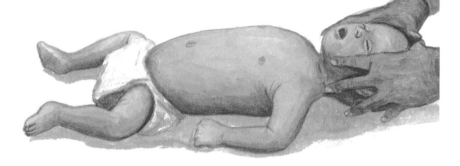

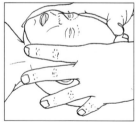

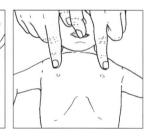

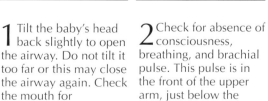

1 Tilt the baby's head back slightly to open the airway. Do not tilt it too far or this may close the airway again. Check the mouth for obstructions.

2 Check for absence of consciousness, breathing, and brachial pulse. This pulse is in the front of the upper arm, just below the main muscle (biceps).

3 Place a fingertip on each nipple. The heart is about midway between them and slightly lower down, towards the base of the breastbone.

❶ If the baby is unconscious, open the airway.

❷ Check that breathing and pulse are absent.

❸ Place two fingers on the lower breastbone.

❹ Give 15 compressions of 1-2 centimetres each, at the rate of 100 per minute,

❺ Alternate with 2 mouth-to-mouth-and-nose inhalations. Stop when the pulse returns.

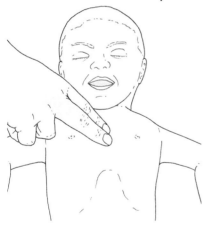

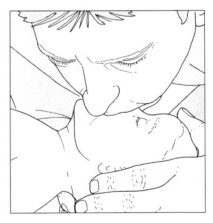

4 Using two fingers, press down about 1-2 centimetres to give one compression. Give 15 at the rate of 100 per minute. Alternate this with 2 inhalations (breaths) of ventilation, using the mouth-to-mouth-and-nose method, step 5.

5 To ventilate, cover the baby's mouth <u>and</u> nose with your mouth, and puff gently — do not blow hard. Check for the brachial pulse every minute. If this returns, stop resuscitation. Keep the baby warm, to prevent chilling.

STABLE SIDE (RECOVERY/COMA) POSITION

The stable side position (recovery or coma position) is for an unconscious casualty, provided there is no risk of neck or back injury (see pages 94, 96).

❶ Lay the casualty on the back, arms in the "surrender" position.

❷ Raise the right knee.

❸ Lock the casualty's right hand with your right hand.

❹ Grasp the casualty's right knee. *continued* ▶

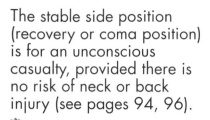

1 An unconscious casualty may choke on fluids or vomit, or roll over dangerously. The stable side position minimizes these risks. First, ensure that there is no risk of a neck or back injury (see pages 94, 96). Gently but firmly, move the casualty to lie flat on his or her back, cradling the head to avoid harm. Straighten the legs, feet slightly apart. Place the arms out and above the head, palms uppermost. Remove keys and other hard objects from the casualty's pockets.

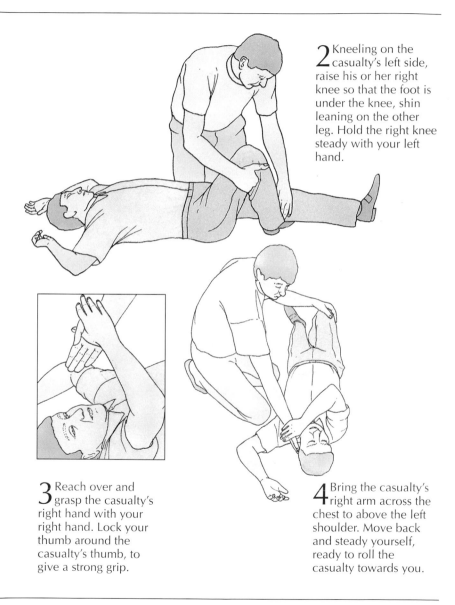

2 Kneeling on the casualty's left side, raise his or her right knee so that the foot is under the knee, shin leaning on the other leg. Hold the right knee steady with your left hand.

3 Reach over and grasp the casualty's right hand with your right hand. Lock your thumb around the casualty's thumb, to give a strong grip.

4 Bring the casualty's right arm across the chest to above the left shoulder. Move back and steady yourself, ready to roll the casualty towards you.

Stable side position *continued*

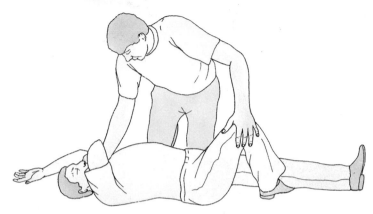

5 Pull on the casualty's knee and arm with your two hands, to roll the casualty towards you. If possible, get another person to help you with this manoeuvre, and to cradle the casualty's head as it turns onto its side. The casualty should not roll right over, but be lying on his or her left side.

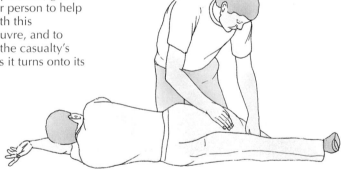

6 Bring the casualty's right arm across and place it out straight, and at an upward angle, so that the forearm touches the chin and the hand is above the level of the top of the head. Move the casualty's right leg so it is slightly bent at the hip and knee, with the right foot on the ground just in front of the left knee.

5 Roll the casualty onto the left side by pulling on the hand and knee.

6 Bring the casualty's right arm and leg out, to act as stabilizers and prevent further rolling.

7 Tip the head slightly so that any fluids or vomit drain away without causing choking.

8 Ensure the casualty is safe and warm, check him or her regularly, and await expert help.

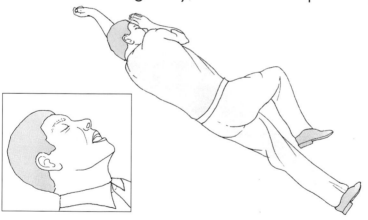

7 Tip the casualty's head back and slightly to the lower side, so that the airway stays open and the tongue cannot flop back and block the throat.

8 In the final stable side position, the casualty lies on the left side, with the right arm and leg out to prevent rolling onto either the back or front. Any fluids or vomit can drain down and out of the mouth, rather than being inhaled into the throat. Check the casualty's condition every 2-3 minutes.

CONTROLLING SEVERE BLEEDING

Like spilt milk, blood from a wound always looks more in quantity than it really is. But if the body loses too much blood, the blood pressure falls, and this endangers the blood supply to the brain and other vital organs. It is essential to stem severe bleeding quickly. ALWAYS use surgical or first-aid gloves if these are available.

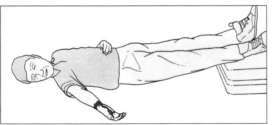 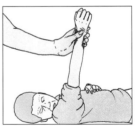

1 The casualty is typically pale and sweating, with obvious blood loss — in this example, from a cut wrist. Blood from an artery is bright red and spurts; blood from a vein is darker red and oozes. The casualty should lie down, feet raised, to concentrate circulating blood in the head and upper body.

2 Wear suitable gloves if available. Elevate (raise) the affected part if possible. This reduces its blood flow, by the effects of gravity, to help slow the blood loss.

1 The casualty lies down with feet raised, to concentrate blood in the head and upper body, where it is most needed.

2 Raise the affected part, so that gravity helps to reduce the blood flow to it. This is called elevation.

3 Press a pad onto the wound for 5-10 minutes, to help it seal. This is called compression.

4 Cover the wound and pad with a dressing.

5 Bandage for protection. Get medical help.

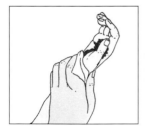 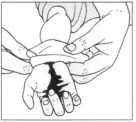 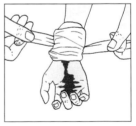

3 Press the wound closed with a clean pad, and maintain the pressure for at least 5 minutes. This helps the blood to begin clotting and slow its escape.

4 When the bleeding has largely stopped, after 10-15 minutes, put another pad onto the site. Do not remove the first one or the bleeding may re-start.

5 Bandage the wound firmly to keep the pads in place and protect against knocks. Get urgent medical help or transport the casualty to hospital.

CHOKING

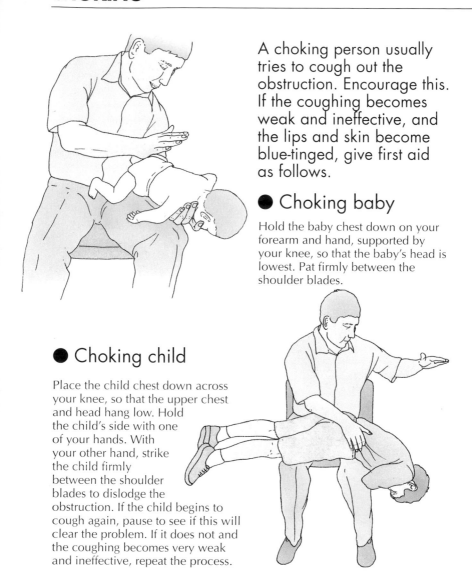

A choking person usually tries to cough out the obstruction. Encourage this. If the coughing becomes weak and ineffective, and the lips and skin become blue-tinged, give first aid as follows.

● Choking baby

Hold the baby chest down on your forearm and hand, supported by your knee, so that the baby's head is lowest. Pat firmly between the shoulder blades.

● Choking child

Place the child chest down across your knee, so that the upper chest and head hang low. Hold the child's side with one of your hands. With your other hand, strike the child firmly between the shoulder blades to dislodge the obstruction. If the child begins to cough again, pause to see if this will clear the problem. If it does not and the coughing becomes very weak and ineffective, repeat the process.

● Choking adult (1)

If the casualty can respond to your request, get him or her to sit in a chair, leaning forward with head just above the knees, supported by the hands. Strike the casualty between the shoulder blades and encourage more coughing.

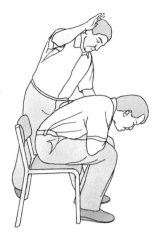

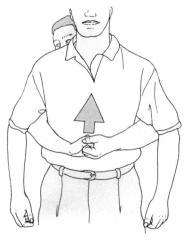

● Choking adult (2)

If there is no response, stand behind the casualty, put your arms around the waist, and lock your hands. Pull upward and inward sharply below the rib cage (Heimlich manoeuvre).

● Choking adult (3)

For an unconscious casualty, kneel astride his or her hips, place the heel of one hand just below the rib cage, place your other hand over this, and push forwards and down.

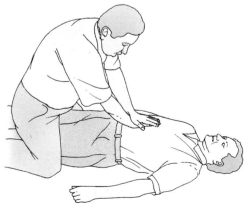

HANGING OR STRANGULATION

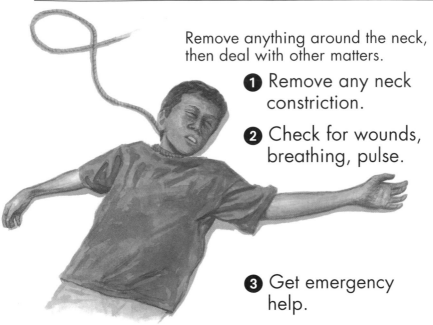

Remove anything around the neck, then deal with other matters.

❶ Remove any neck constriction.

❷ Check for wounds, breathing, pulse.

❸ Get emergency help.

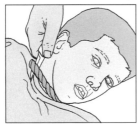
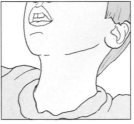
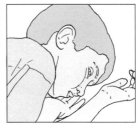

1 Cut the rope or other constriction, slicing <u>away</u> from the neck. Do not waste time trying to undo knots (and these may be required by the authorities as evidence).

2 Check the neck for punctures or deep wounds, and deal with these. Check breathing and pulse. If these are absent, resuscitate as required (see page 28).

3 When the casualty is breathing, put him or her in the stable side position (see page 40). Get medical help as soon as possible and also inform the police.

SUFFOCATION

The casualty may be unconscious with pale, even blue-tinged skin.

❶ Make sure your actions will cause no further harm.

❷ Remove any object causing the suffocation.

❸ Check breathing and pulse.

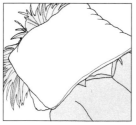

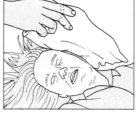

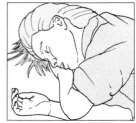

1 Quickly assess the situation. Ensure that you will not cause harm when removing the cause of suffocation, for example, by letting the casualty fall.

2 Remove the cause of the suffocation — in this case, a pillow. For a plastic bag, cut it away. Check breathing and pulse, and resuscitate as required (see page 28)

3 When the casualty is breathing, put him or her in the stable side position (see page 40). Get medical help. In suspicious cases, also inform the police.

DROWNING

A casualty who has been rescued from drowning, or who has inhaled any water, should always receive hospital attention.

❶ Check pulse and breathing, resuscitate, and keep warm.

❷ Monitor the condition, get the casualty to hospital.

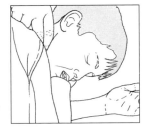

1 Check breathing and pulse. If these are absent, resuscitate as required (see page 28). When breathing and pulse are re-started, place the casualty in the stable side position (see page 40). Remove wet clothing but make sure the casualty is kept covered and warm. Get emergency help. Keep watch for vomiting.

2 Check the pulse every minute or two, and reassure the casualty. Ensure that he or she receives medical attention, due to danger of lung infection

GAS INHALATION

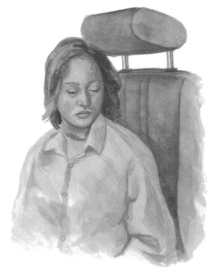

This may happen with vehicle exhaust fumes or defective gas appliances, or at an industrial workplace.

1 Ventilate the area. Get in and out fast.

2 Check breathing and pulse.

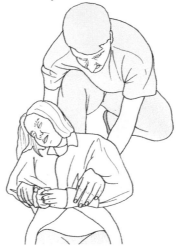

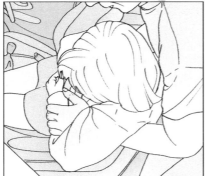

1 Open doors and windows to disperse the gas, such as carbon monoxide from a vehicle exhaust, which causes a characteristic red-faced appearance. Turn off the gas source. Do not be overcome yourself — plan your movements.

2 Get the casualty into fresh air. Check breathing and pulse, and resuscitate as required (see page 28). When breathing and pulse are re-started, place in the stable side position (see page 40). Arrange urgent transport to hospital.

SMOKE INHALATION

The casualty may have singed hair and sooted skin, and be coughing or unconscious.

1 Get the casualty clear. Check breathing and pulse, resuscitate.

2 Give oxygen if available, get help.

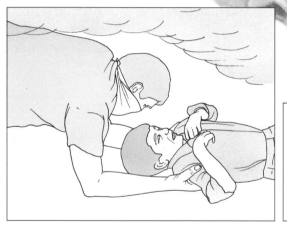

1 Be aware of your own safety. Is there another door or window for better access and escape? Keep low to avoid inhaling smoke, and cover your mouth and nose with a wet cloth. Pull the casualty clear, into fresh air if possible. Check breathing and pulse, resuscitate as necessary (see page 28).

2 Give oxygen if available, following equipment instructions. Ensure urgent hospital treatment due to risk of delayed burn reactions in the airway and lungs.

SEVERE ASTHMA ATTACK

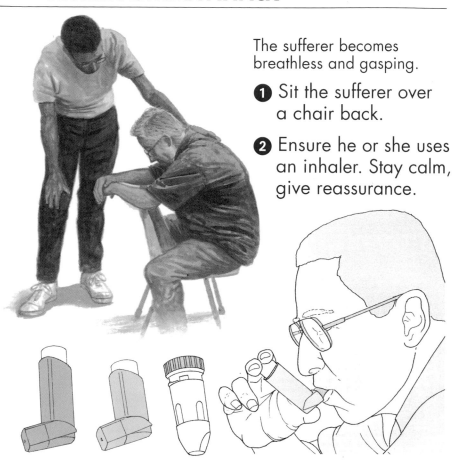

The sufferer becomes breathless and gasping.

❶ Sit the sufferer over a chair back.

❷ Ensure he or she uses an inhaler. Stay calm, give reassurance.

1 Sit the sufferer facing a chair back, leaning on it to ease breathing. Open a nearby door or window for fresh air. To aid breathing, loosen tight clothing around the neck, chest, and abdomen. Keep onlookers away.

2 Locate the sufferer's inhaler, or ask if another person has a similar one. Use it as prescribed. You can help greatly by staying calm and offering reassurance, since the sufferer's worry and panic tend to worsen the condition.

HEART ATTACK

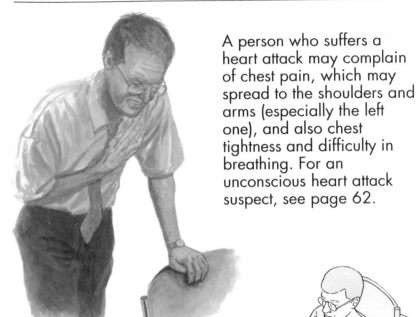

A person who suffers a heart attack may complain of chest pain, which may spread to the shoulders and arms (especially the left one), and also chest tightness and difficulty in breathing. For an unconscious heart attack suspect, see page 62.

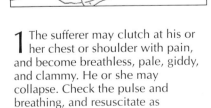

1 The sufferer may clutch at his or her chest or shoulder with pain, and become breathless, pale, giddy, and clammy. He or she may collapse. Check the pulse and breathing, and resuscitate as required (see page 28).

2 If the sufferer is conscious, prop him or her on cushions, with knees raised. Loosen tight clothing and reassure the sufferer. At the earliest opportunity, call for emergency help and describe the possibility of heart attack.

1 Observe the signs and symptoms. Check pulse and breathing, resuscitate if necessary.

2 Call for emergency help. Make the sufferer comfortable.

3 Monitor the sufferer, give reassurance.

4 Give appropriate medication, such as angina tablets. Await emergency help.

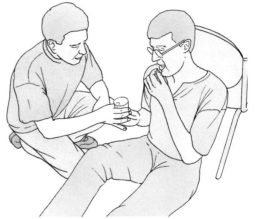

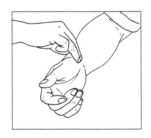

3 Check the sufferer's pulse and general condition every few minutes. Open windows to allow in fresh air. Stay calm and keep onlookers away.

4 If the sufferer has suitable medication, such as angina tablets, he or she should take this according to the directions. It may help to give an aspirin either in a glass of water or dissolved in the mouth. Note the sufferer's condition and progress, so you can inform the ambulance or medical staff when they arrive.

SHOCK

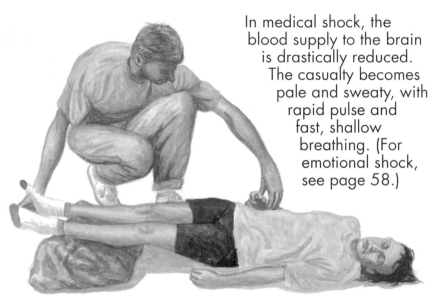

In medical shock, the blood supply to the brain is drastically reduced. The casualty becomes pale and sweaty, with rapid pulse and fast, shallow breathing. (For emotional shock, see page 58.)

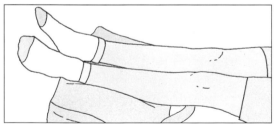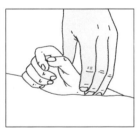

1 Try to find the cause of shock. It may be severe blood loss from a wound (external or internal) or ulcer, fluid loss by copious vomiting or diarrhoea, severe allergic reaction, blood poisoning, or cardiogenic causes such as a heart attack. Deal with the cause if possible. Raise the casualty's legs and feet.

2 Call for emergency help in any way you can. Check the casualty's pulse every 2-3 minutes. Pass on this information when help arrives.

❶ Assess the casualty's symptoms and try to determine the cause of shock. Deal with this if possible. Raise the casualty's legs and feet.

❷ Ensure emergency help is on its way. Take the casualty's pulse.

❸ Keep the casualty warm but not hot. Give reassurance but nothing by mouth.

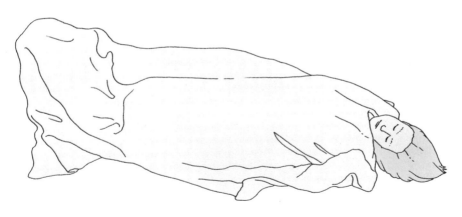

3 Cover the casualty to keep him or her warm but not too hot. Give reassurance and monitor the casualty's condition, but do not let the casualty eat or drink anything. The raised legs should ensure that as much blood as possible reaches the brain.

FAINTING

A faint can be due to emotional shock, fatigue, hunger, warm humid surroundings, or various medical conditions.

● Make the casualty comfortable, raise the feet, check for injury, reassure, and arrange for a medical check.

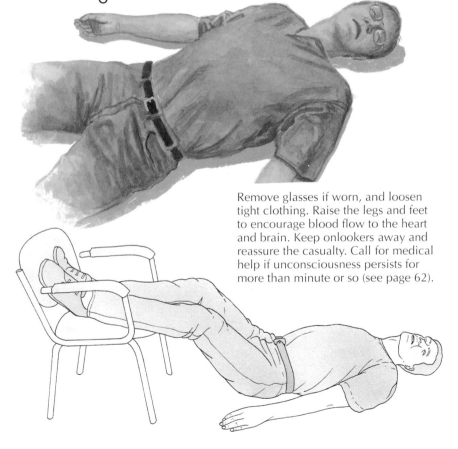

Remove glasses if worn, and loosen tight clothing. Raise the legs and feet to encourage blood flow to the heart and brain. Keep onlookers away and reassure the casualty. Call for medical help if unconsciousness persists for more than minute or so (see page 62).

FITS (CONVULSIONS OR SEIZURES)

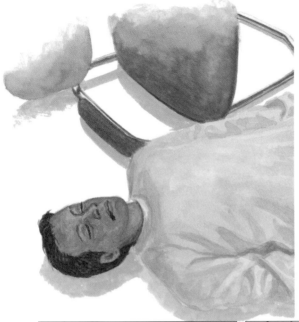

Most fits are due to an underlying condition such as epilepsy (see also page 60).

❶ Clear the area to prevent injury to the sufferer.

❷ Get medical help, keep the sufferer safe.

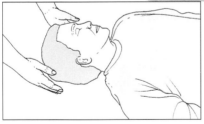

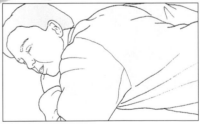

1 The sufferer may go rigid or make jerky movements, have blood in the mouth from a bitten lip or tongue, and lose bowel or bladder control. Clear the area. Guide the head to prevent injury, but do not restrain the sufferer.

2 Do not put anything in the sufferer's mouth. Allow the fit to progress. As it subsides, put the sufferer in the stable side position (see page 40), give reassurance, and keep onlookers away. Arrange for urgent medical attention.

FEBRILE FITS (FEVER CONVULSIONS)

This condition may occur in the very young, usually due to a high body temperature from an infection.

① Remove coverings, cool the baby, wrap in light clothing.

② Take the baby to a hospital or medical centre, monitoring his or her condition.

DO NOT over-wrap babies in warm conditions.

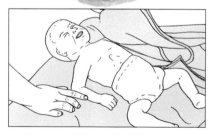

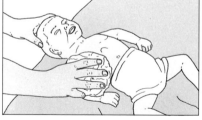

1 The baby is usually feverish, and may roll its eyes and make jerky limb movements. Take off blankets and clothing. Sponge the baby with tepid (not cold) water, to reduce the body temperature gradually.

2 Give reassurance, especially to the parents — this type of fit looks more serious than it usually is. When the baby is recovering, wrap in light clothing, and take him or her to a local hospital or medical centre for an examination.

CONCUSSION

This is temporary loss of consciousness due to a knock or blow on the head. The casualty should always have a medical check.

1 Make the casualty comfortable, keep him or her still and quiet.

2 Arrange for transport to hospital.

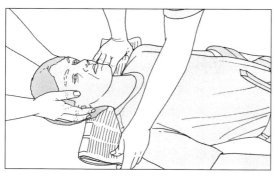

1 Check the casualty's pulse and breathing, and resuscitate if necessary (see page 28). Examine for head injury (see pages 70, 93). The casualty may seem agitated and confused on recovery, so give reassurance and keep onlookers away. If you need to move him or her, improvize a neck collar (see page 96).

2 Get emergency medical help. Keep the casualty warm, in the stable side position if necessary (see page 40). Always ensure an examination in hospital.

UNCONSCIOUSNESS

If you find someone unconscious, or a person collapses and loses consciousness, there are dozens of possible causes — from a temporary faint due to hunger or fatigue, to a heart attack or stroke (see pages 54, 64). The situation may provide clues to the cause, such as an empty pill bottle indicating a drug overdose; consult the relevant pages. Attend to the casualty's priorities and get urgent medical help at the earliest opportunity (see pages 12, 16).

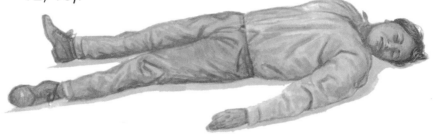

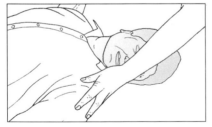

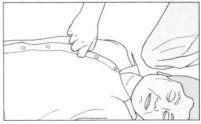

1 After checking the area is safe, approach the casualty and assess the situation for a possible cause. Speak to the casualty first, to assess verbal response (see page 17). If there is none, shake the shoulder gently to assess physical response.

2 If there is no reaction, assess response to pain, by pinching his or her fingernail, or rubbing your knuckle on the breastbone. Check the pulse and breathing, resuscitate if necessary (see page 28). Get urgent medical help.

1 Approach carefully in case of danger, such as invisible fumes. Speak to the casualty and shake the shoulders, to assess the level of response (see page 17).

2 If necessary, check response to pain, and check pulse and breathing. Resuscitate as necessary. Arrange for medical assistance.

3 Regularly monitor the casualty's condition.

4 Put the casualty in the stable side position, examine for a possible cause of the unconsciousness, and wait for assistance.

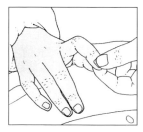 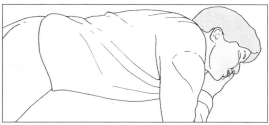

3 After another few seconds, re-check the response to pain with a finger pinch. The casualty may be roused by this stimulus. Monitor the condition.

4 If the casualty does not respond, put him or her in the stable side position (see page 40). Place the right hand under the chin to keep the airway open. Keep a check on the pulse and breathing. Carry out an examination for the possible cause (see page 17). Stay with the casualty until expert help arrives.

SUSPECTED STROKE

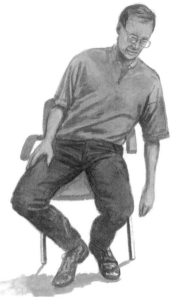

Signs of a stroke (blockage of the blood supply to the brain) include a red face, drooling, loss of muscle control, and paralysis.

❶ Check the signs and symptoms.

❷ Lay the sufferer down, loosen tight clothing, get help.

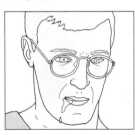

1 The sufferer may appear red-faced and dribbling, with loss of balance and muscle control, and paralysis, often of one side of the body.

2 If the sufferer is conscious, get help to lay him or her down, head raised. Loosen clothing. Call for emergency medical help. Stay with the sufferer and give reassurance. If he or she is unconscious, put in the stable side position (see page 40). Monitor pulse and breathing (see page 28).

PART THREE

BLEEDING AND WOUNDS

OBJECT EMBEDDED IN A WOUND

Cleaning small pieces of gravel and similar items from a wound is part of routine first aid. But if a large object is embedded in a wound, such as a knife, or a shard of glass or metal, this should be left in place while emergency help is obtained and the wound is dressed. Removing the object could worsen bleeding.

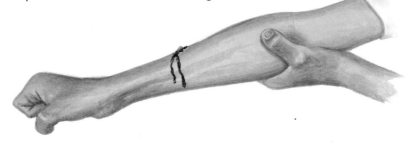

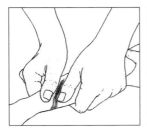

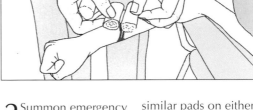

1 Squeeze the sides of the wound together and maintain pressure to slow the bleeding. Do not remove the object unless it falls out naturally.

2 Summon emergency help as soon as you can. Maintain pressure for 10 minutes, with the part raised to slow blood escape. Place rolled-up bandages or similar pads on either side of the object so that they are higher than the object. This prevents direct pressure on the object as the wound is dressed.

❶ Apply pressure to close the wound and reduce bleeding (see page 44). Do not remove the object.

❷ Summon emergency help. Maintain pressure for 10 minutes. Pad around the wound and object to prevent pressure on the object.

❸ Cover the wound and pads with thick dressings and bandage in place.

❹ Keep the part still and protected from knocks.

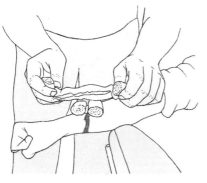

3 Place a thick wad of dressing or other clean material over the pads. Bandage this in place, avoiding direct pressure on the embedded object.

4 Build up the bandage with plenty of turns, and finish off with tape or a knot well away from the object. Keep the part still while obtaining expert help.

OBJECT IN EYE

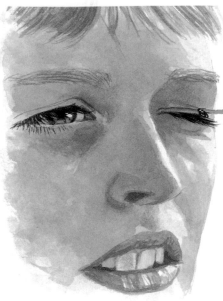

Do not remove an object impaled in or near the eye (see page 73). Apply a dressing and get hospital attention.

❶ Pad the wound. Avoid pressure on the object.

❷ Bandage both eyes.

❸ Take to hospital.

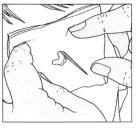

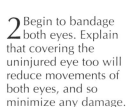

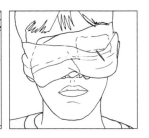

1 Apply a dressing, but avoid pressure on the object. Cut a hole in the pad, or put pads around the object, or place a cup over it, to relieve direct pressure.

2 Begin to bandage both eyes. Explain that covering the uninjured eye too will reduce movements of both eyes, and so minimize any damage.

3 Put a bandage around the head, over both eyes. Talk to and reassure the casualty (sounds will be very important). Take the casualty to hospital.

OBJECT IN EAR

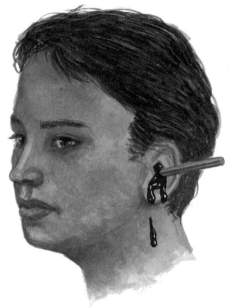

Do not remove an object impaled in or near the ear. Apply a dressing and get the casualty to a hospital or medical centre.

❶ Pad the wound, avoiding direct pressure on the object.

❷ Bandage the area.

❸ Take to hospital.

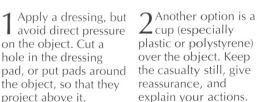

1 Apply a dressing, but avoid direct pressure on the object. Cut a hole in the dressing pad, or put pads around the object, so that they project above it.

2 Another option is a cup (especially plastic or polystyrene) over the object. Keep the casualty still, give reassurance, and explain your actions.

3 When the object is protected from direct pressure, apply a bandage, strap, or tape to secure the protection in position. Get the casualty to hospital.

CUTS ON HEAD

CAUTION: With a head wound, check for signs of serious head or neck injury (see pages 93, 96) and take appropriate action. Facial and scalp wounds tend to bleed profusely since the skin has a rich blood supply.

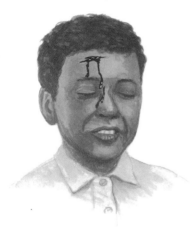

❶ Wash the wound. Press the edges.

❷ Maintain pressure to slow bleeding.

❸ Position dressing.

❹ Bandage in place.

❺ Secure so bandage cannot slip.

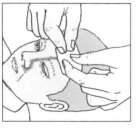 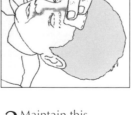 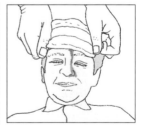

1 Quickly wash dirt from the wound with clean water. Apply a dressing and pinch the wound's edges together to close the gap and reduce blood leakage.

2 Maintain this pressure for 10 minutes. When the bleeding has slowed, leave the first dressing in place, and apply a second over it.

3 Position one end of a roller bandage over the dressings and begin to bandage around the head, holding the dressings in place with one hand.

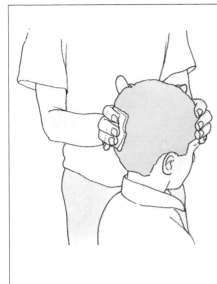

CUT ON THE BACK OF THE HEAD

Follow the main stages as described below. To apply pressure on the wound and reduce bleeding, especially when the cut is under the hair, hold a dressing on the cut with one hand and place your other hand on the casualty's forehead. Press your hands together to help close the cut, for about 10 minutes.

Apply a second dressing over the first and bandage firmly over both as shown in steps 3-5, with offset turns so that the bandage cannot slip up or down. Get the casualty to a hospital or medical centre.

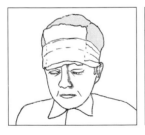

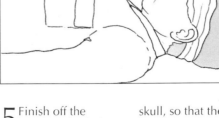

4 Continue bandaging and gradually work the turns up and down the back of the head (if the cut is at the front), for stability and to prevent slippage.

5 Finish off the bandage firmly but not too tightly. Ensure that, for a front head cut, some turns of the bandage are below the rear-facing dome of the skull, so that the bandage cannot slip up or down. Take the casualty to a hospital or medical centre.

NOSEBLEED

This problem has numerous causes, from a physical knock, to sneezing or blowing the nose hard.

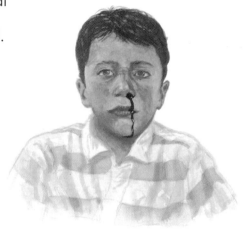

1 Apply a pad to the nose.

2 Press the pad for 10 minutes. Do not tip the head back.

3 If bleeding re-starts, repeat.

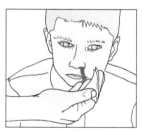 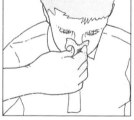 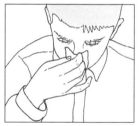

1 Ask the casualty to keep his or her head upright. Place a large pad over the nostrils and squeeze this to apply pressure and slow the bleeding.

2 Maintain pressure for 10 minutes. The casualty should lean forwards, or he or she may swallow blood and feel sick. Remove the pad carefully.

3 If bleeding continues, repeat steps 1-2. When the nosebleed has stopped, the casualty should not blow or rub the nose for several hours.

CUT ON OR NEAR EYE

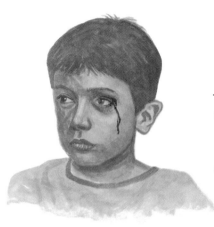

The eye's ceaseless movements can worsen the effects of a cut. Since both eyes usually move together, it may be advisable to cover both eyes.

❶ Steady the casualty's head, and reassure.

❷ Place a pad over the injured eye. Bandage both eyes.

❸ Get expert help.

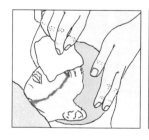

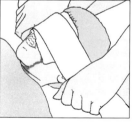

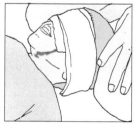

1 Put the casualty's head between your knees to keep it still. Place a light pad over the injured eye. Talk to the casualty and explain what you are doing.

2 For an object in the wound (see page 68), put pads beside it or a cup over it, to relieve direct pressure of the bandage. Begin to bandage both eyes.

3 Cover both eyes so the injured eye does not move with the uncovered eye. Stay with the casualty and give reassurance until expert help arrives.

CUT LIP

The lips have a rich blood and nerve supply. When cut, they may be painful and bleed profusely — but they also heal quickly.

❶ Clean and apply a pad, with a finger under the lip. Do not tip the head back

❷ Press for 10 minutes, dress, and get medical help.

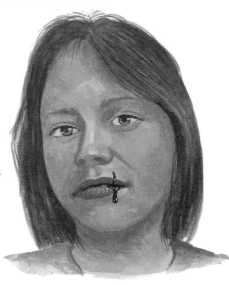

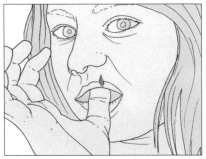

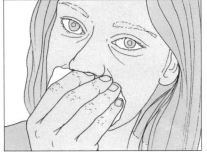

1 Remove any dirt and clean the wound. The casualty places a finger or thumb under the lip at the site of the cut. Put a pad on the cut, and press this for 5-10 minutes. Ask the casualty to sit forward so the blood drips away.

2 If the cut continues to bleed, do not remove the pad. Put another pad over it. This area is difficult to bandage, so you may need to keep the pads applied by hand. Keep the casualty calm and quiet, and take him or her for medical attention.

BROKEN OR LOST TOOTH

A knocked-out tooth can sometimes stay alive and re-implant itself, if replaced quickly in its socket. Or it may be re-attached by modern dental methods.

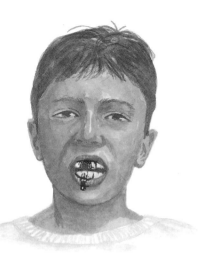

1 If the tooth is found, dip it in milk and replace it in the socket.

2 If not, press a pad on the empty socket.

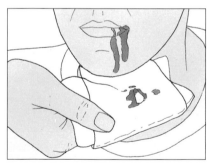

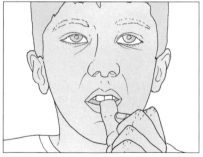

1 The casualty should lean forwards so that blood drips away. If the tooth has come out fairly cleanly, with some or all of its root, dip it in milk and push it back into the socket. Do not try to clean the tooth.

2 Hold the replaced tooth in position until expert help is available. If the tooth cannot be replaced, the casualty should have a mouth rinse, hold a pad over the socket, and go to a dentist, hospital, or medical centre.

CUT PALM OF HAND

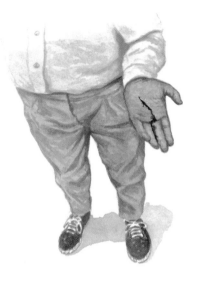

An incision or penetrating cut on the palm requires careful dressing, or the wound will re-open and gape, which slows healing.

❶ Wash and cover with a pad.

❷ Press the cut closed for 10 minutes.

❸ Clench fingers on a second dressing pad, and bandage.

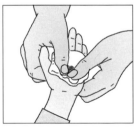 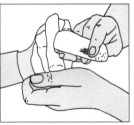 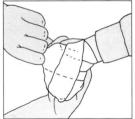

1 Wash the area under cool running water so it is clean. Cover it with sterile gauze, or a similar pad or dressing, and then firmly press the skin to close the cut.

2 Raise the hand to reduce blood flow and keep pressing the cut closed for 10 minutes. Put a second pad on the first. Clench the fingers over it.

3 Secure the second pad and clenched fingers in place with a bandage. Obtain medical advice for gaping cuts or if there are signs of infection.

CUT FINGER

Most cuts and other wounds on the finger are not serious, and are easily cleaned or dressed. However, if the cut is large or deep enough to damage muscles and tendons, so that finger or hand movements are affected, seek expert help.

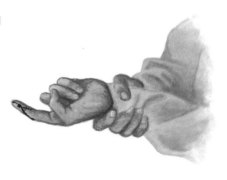

1 Wash and apply a dressing.

2 Apply pressure for 10 minutes.

3 Put on a second dressing, and cover.

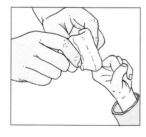 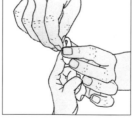 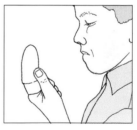

1 Wash the cut under cool running water so it is clean. Cover it with sterile gauze or a similar pad or dressing, and then firmly press the cut closed.

2 Raise the finger to reduce blood flow, while pressing the cut closed for about 10 minutes. Put a second pad over the first to secure it.

3 Secure the second dressing in place with sticking plaster, tape, or similar. Obtain medical advice for gaping cuts or if there are signs of infection.

PENETRATING CHEST WOUND

If a wound penetrates into the chest cavity, this may allow air to enter the space between the inside of the rib cage and the lungs, and lead to a pneumo-thorax or collapsed lung. This will cause great difficulty in breathing. Obtain emergency help as soon as possible, and try to keep the casualty still.

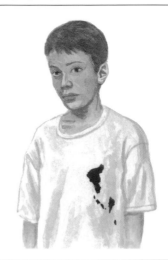

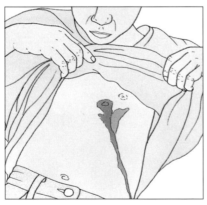

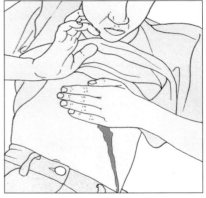

1 Get the casualty to sit down, stay calm, and breathe slowly, since panting or deep breathing may worsen the condition. Ask him or her to lean over to the wounded side, while you assess the extent of the wound.

2 Ask the casualty to place his or her hand flat over the wound. This helps to reduce bleeding and also prevents air from entering the chest through the wound, which would cause a sucking sound and possibly lead to lung collapse.

1 The casualty should sit down, lean to the injured side, and stay still.

2 Encourage the casualty to place his or her hand over the wound, to control bleeding.

3 Put a plastic covering (clean plastic bag or similar) over the wound.

4 Then cover with an adhesive dressing or tape. Get emergency medical help.

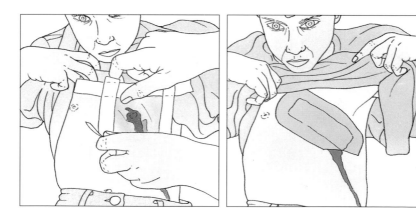

3 Put a piece of plastic (from a clean plastic bag or similar) over the wound. Leave one corner loose, to allow air to escape as the casualty exhales. If possible, tape the sheet in place with adhesive tape, or use a large roller bandage.

4 Cover the wound and sheet with a large adhesive dressing. Again, cut a corner from this, so exhaled air can escape from the wound. In the meantime, call for urgent medical help. Keep the casualty still and calm until medical help arrives.

ABDOMINAL WOUND

A casualty with a large abdominal wound should lie down with knees raised and keep still, while you call for emergency help. Cover and dress the wound while waiting for assistance.

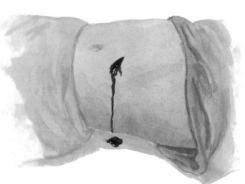

1 Lay the casualty down, with legs raised.

2 Cover and tape or bandage the wound.

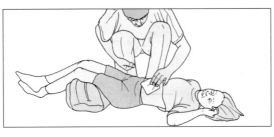

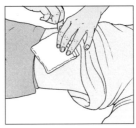

1 Get the casualty to lie down. Prop up his or her knees on an object, to minimize the stretching of the skin and muscles in the abdominal wall (abdominal tension). Call for emergency help at the first opportunity. Keep the casualty still and quiet, while you stay calm and offer reassurance.

2 Apply a dressing pad and secure it with adhesive tape or a large bandage. Do not move the casualty. Wait for help.

CUT KNEE

The cut knee benefits from being well bandaged, to keep the leg straight during healing.

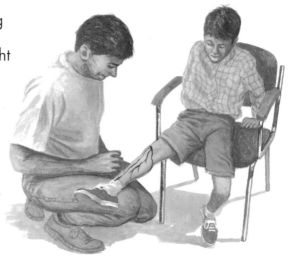

1 Clean the cut.

2 Apply pad and pressure.

3 Bandage securely.

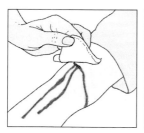
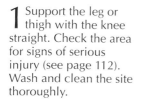

1 Support the leg or thigh with the knee straight. Check the area for signs of serious injury (see page 112). Wash and clean the site thoroughly.

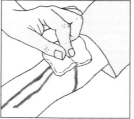

2 Apply a clean, dry pad to the site and press the cut closed with your fingers for 10 minutes. If necessary, put a second pad over the first.

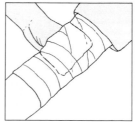

3 Place a bandage over the pad and make secure turns on, above, and below the knee. This keeps the knee straight to encourage healing.

BLEEDING VARICOSE VEIN

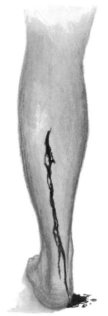

Varicose veins are a medical condition in which veins become swollen and engorged with blood. This can occur anywhere in the body, but it is most commonly seen in the lower legs. If a varicose vein is knocked, cut, or over-stretched, it may split and bleed profusely. Treat as for other cuts, with pressure and dressing, and seek medical advice.

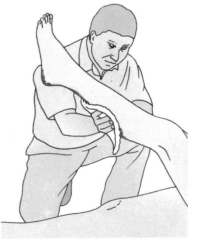

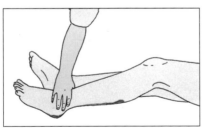

1 Ask the casualty to lie down in a quiet place. Ask onlookers to move away. Prepare to raise or elevate the affected leg, using an object as a support.

2 Lift the affected leg to slow blood flow, and press a large pad onto the wound. Keep this in place and maintain pressure for at least 10 minutes.

❶ Ask the casualty to lie down in a quiet place where you can give first aid undisturbed.

❷ Raise the affected part. Place a large, clean pad over the area and maintain pressure to slow the bleeding.

❸ Add further pads as necessary, keeping the part raised.

❹ Bandage firmly and obtain medical advice.

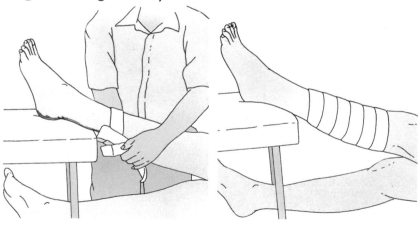

3 Meanwhile, support the raised leg with a chair or similar object. If the first pad becomes blood-soaked, put a second one over it. Bandage them in place.

4 Bandage the leg firmly and keep it raised for as long as possible. Obtain medical help since the varicose veins may need expert attention.

SEVERED OR AMPUTATED PART

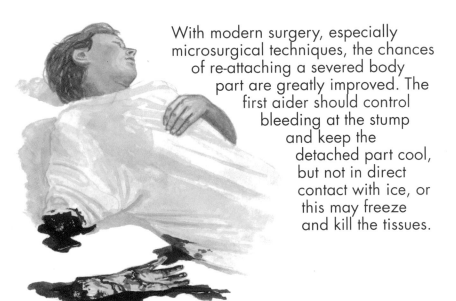

With modern surgery, especially microsurgical techniques, the chances of re-attaching a severed body part are greatly improved. The first aider should control bleeding at the stump and keep the detached part cool, but not in direct contact with ice, or this may freeze and kill the tissues.

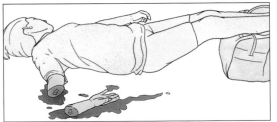

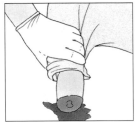

1 The casualty should lie down with feet raised, to concentrate blood in the head and body. Monitor breathing and pulse, and resuscitate if necessary (see page 28). Arrange for emergency medical help or transport at the earliest opportunity. (Be aware of the risks of infection from blood, see page 10.)

2 Slow bleeding by locating and compressing the main artery (blood vessel) or arteries in the stump. In this example, it is the arm's brachial artery.

❶ Lay the casualty down, feet raised. Get medical help as soon as possible, or prepare to transport the casualty and part.

❷ Try to control bleeding at the stump by pressure on the artery just above the wound.

❸ Place plenty of padding over the stump.

❹ Apply dressings, bandage in place, and raise the affected part if possible.

❺ Keep the part cool but <u>not</u> frozen, such as in a sealed bag, in another bag and in iced water. Get help or transport to hospital.

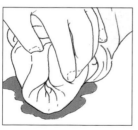 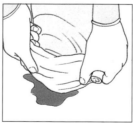 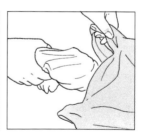

3 Place rolls of padding around any exposed bones or other hard tissues, to reduce direct pressure on them when the dressing is applied.

4 Apply plenty of pads and dressings over the wounded area. If bleeding persists, put more pads on top of them. Secure by bandages or tapes.

5 Put the severed part in a clean plastic bag or similar. Keep it cool by putting it near (but <u>not</u> in direct contact with) chilled or iced water. Take to hospital.

KNIFE WOUNDS

Do not attempt to remove an embedded knife or other weapon. Get medical help at the first opportunity. Pad the area for protection and to reduce blood loss, and keep the casualty calm and still while waiting.

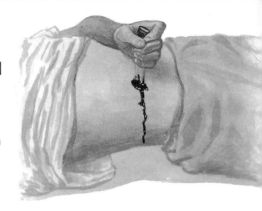

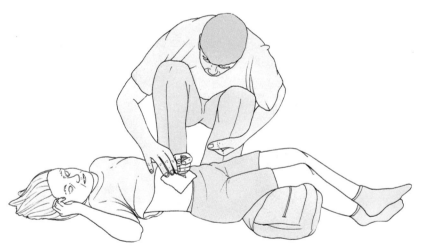

1 Call for medical help as soon as you can. Get the casualty to lie down in a position that takes the strain and tension off the wound site. For example, with an abdominal knife wound, the casualty's legs should be raised to reduce stretching of the abdominal wall. Leave the knife or other weapon in the wound; removing it could cause further damage. Clean around the area. Reassure the casualty that help is coming, and keep him or her still and quiet.

1 At the first opportunity, call for emergency medical help. Get the casualty to lie down in a posture than minimizes stretching and tension around the wounded area.

2 Place pads around the wound, to apply pressure and slow bleeding, and to stabilize the knife. Do not attempt to remove the knife.

3 Tape or bandage the pads. Monitor the casualty, give reassurance, wait for help.

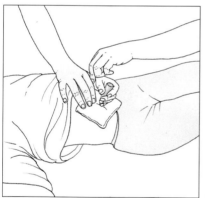

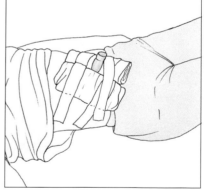

2 Place rolls, padding, and other items around the area so that when it is taped or bandaged, these will compress the wound and help to close it, thereby reducing blood loss. But do not put direct pressure on the knife.

3 Strap, tape, or bandage the padding in place, so the wound is pressed closed and the knife is stabilized. If the injured part is a limb, raise it to reduce blood flow. Stay with the casualty, who should keep still, until help arrives.

BULLET WOUNDS

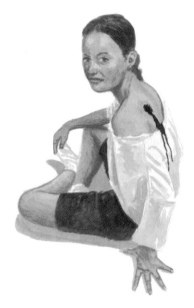

The typical pistol or rifle bullet causes a small entry wound. Flash marks indicate a close-range shot. The bullet may pass through the body tissues and out through an exit hole, which is larger and shows more tissue and skin damage. The bullet may cause internal wounding and bleeding which is not immediately obvious to the observer.

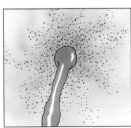

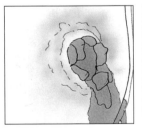

1 The entry wound is typically small and "neat". Flash burns indicate a close-range shot (important police medical evidence). The exit wound, if present, is usually larger, with more tissue disruption and bleeding. Treat this first, especially if it is in the chest. Call for emergency medical help.

INTERNAL DAMAGE

A bullet may not travel in a straight line through the body. It can be deflected by bones and other hard parts, causing further internal damage, and then emerge at a different angle. Monitor the casualty's breathing and pulse at all times (see page 28).

1 Ensure there is no further danger. Call for medical help as soon as you can. Quickly examine the casualty to locate the wounds.

2 Place a pad, plastic sheet, or adhesive plaster over the exit wound. Secure in place.

3 Repeat for the entry wound. Keep the casualty still, monitor pulse and breathing (see page 28), treat for shock (see page 56).

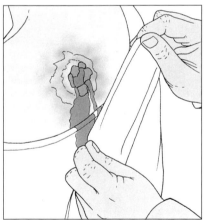

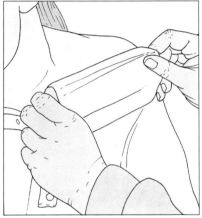

2 Place a large pad or adhesive plaster over the exit wound, to reduce blood loss and possibility of infection. In the chest, cover the wound with an airtight sheet such as a piece of plastic (see page 78). Secure the coverings in place.

3 Treat the entry wound in a similar way. Get the casualty into a comfortable position, and keep him or her still and quiet. Monitor pulse and breathing; treat for shock. If the bullet is available, pass it to the authorities.

SHOTGUN WOUNDS

A shotgun fires a spray of small pellets called shot, which may enter the body to different depths.

① Remove surface pellets, leave embedded ones.

② Dress the wound, take the casualty for medical help.

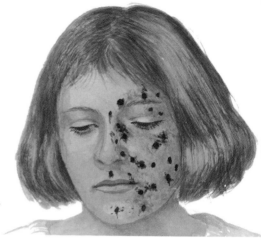

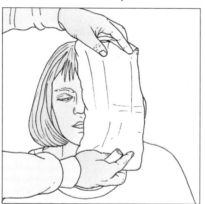

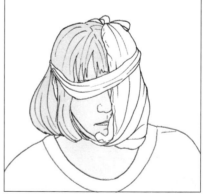

1 Quickly examine the casualty to assess the extent of the wounds. Pellets are unlikely to reach deep organs, but be aware of this possibility. Remove loose pellets; do not try to prise out deep ones. Cover the area with a large pad.

2 Tape, bandage, or strap the dressing pad in place, but not too tightly. Ensure the casualty can see and breathe. However if one eye is wounded, cover both eyes to reduce their movements (see page 73). Get hospital attention.

PART FOUR

FRACTURES AND DISLOCATIONS

PRINCIPLES OF TREATMENT

WHAT ARE FRACTURES AND DISLOCATIONS?

A fracture is a break in a bone. There are various types. A greenstick fracture is a crack or incomplete break, as in a bendy bush branch; it usually occurs in younger children, whose bones are flexible. In a closed fracture, the skin over the site is not broken, and the risk of infection is limited. In an open fracture (see page 114), the skin is broken and the tissues and bone ends may protrude; the risk of infection is high. A simple fracture means the main damage is to the bone itself. Complicated fractures involve damage to other tissues, such as nerves and blood vessels.

A dislocation happens in a joint. The bone ends, which normally move smoothly over each other, come apart. When a joint is wrenched or over-flexed, with ligament damage but no proper dislocation, this is usually called a sprain (see page 152).

It may be difficult for the first aider to distinguish between sprains, dislocations, and fractures. In most cases, this is not vital, since the general actions are the same — call for emergency medical help, and follow the treatment guidelines below. Consider making splints and other more complex treatments only if medical help will be delayed, or if the casualty has to be transported some distance.

1 Examine the casualty to assess the extent of the injury. Note pain at rest or on movement, tenderness, swelling, deformity (compare the opposing uninjured part), open wounds, numbness, reduced movement, or paralysis.

2 Arrange emergency medical help as soon as possible. Make the casualty comfortable, reassure, and deal with wounds and bleeding. Monitor pulse and breathing, and resuscitate if necessary (see page 28).

3 Stabilize injured parts against further movement, with items such as pads, blankets, belts, bandages, sticks, cushions, and so on. "Bind as you find" (see page 106). Beware of shock (see page 56) due to internal bleeding.

FRACTURED SKULL

Move the casualty to the stable side position, but beware of the possibility of neck injury (see page 96).

❶ Check the casualty for injuries. Send for medical help. Apply a neck collar.

❷ Dress wounds, put in a stable position.

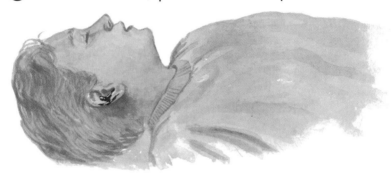

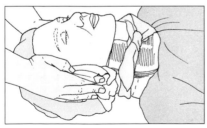 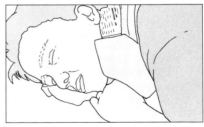

1 Signs of skull fracture include bruises on the head, wounds and bleeding, and blood or clearish fluid (cerebrospinal fluid) oozing from the ear. Call for emergency help as soon as possible. Apply a neck collar (see page 96) before moving the casualty.

2 Carefully but quickly, dress any wounds with pads and tape or bandages (see page 70). Move the casualty carefully to the stable side position (see page 40), with the injured side lowest. Monitor pulse and breathing, and give reassurance.

SUSPECTED BACK INJURY

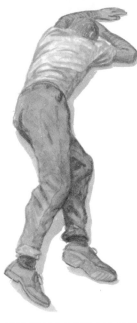

DO NOT move a casualty with a suspected back injury, unless his or her life is in danger (see page 96).

❶ Get emergency medical help. Keep the casualty warm, and reassure.

❷ Assess the extent of the injuries.

❸ If necessary, roll the casualty over like a log.

❹ Keep the airway clear, monitor pulse and breathing.

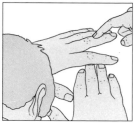

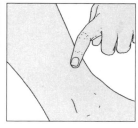

1 Call for emergency medical help as soon as possible. If the casualty is conscious, ask him or her to lie still and quiet, and reassure that help is on the way.

2 Assess the degree of injury by checking feeling and movement in the limbs (see right). Check pulse and breathing, resuscitate if necessary (see page 28).

SIGNS OF INJURY
Ask the casualty if he or she can feel anything as you press in turn on each arm, hand, ankle, and toe. Ask the casualty to move these same parts, in turn. Relate your findings to the medical staff when they arrive. Keep the casualty warm and still, and give reassurance.

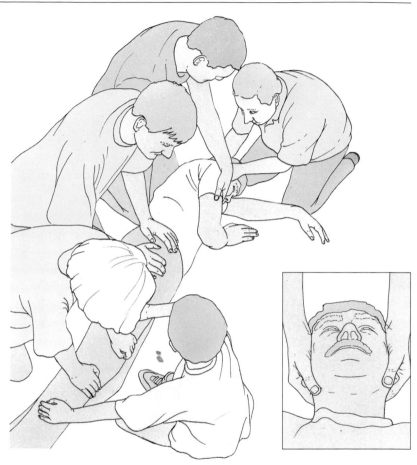

3 If it is absolutely necessary to move the casualty, improvize a neck collar (see page 96) to keep the head steady and so minimize further damage to the neck. Roll the casualty over like a log, with the help of others if available, trying to keep the neck and back in the same relative positions.

4 Monitor the casualty's condition while waiting. If there are breathing problems, lift the casualty's chin slightly by holding the sides of the head.

SUSPECTED NECK INJURY

Follow the actions for suspected back injury (see page 94). In general, DO NOT move a casualty with any possible spinal injury, unless his or her life is in danger. Movement may cause further, permanent damage.

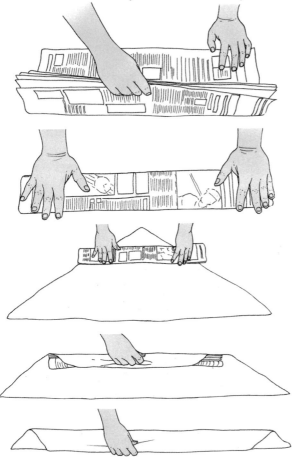

1 The neck collar supports and stabilizes the casualty's neck position while waiting for medical help to arrive, and is vital should moving the casualty become essential. Use magazines, thick textiles, a newspaper (as here), or any similar supporting material. Fold the sheets into a long strip about 8-12 centimetres wide.

2 Roll up the strip in a triangular bandage, scarf, towel, or similar item. This should form a fairly stiff central section with two loose ends. One helper can be preparing the neck collar while the senior first aider attends to the casualty's condition and determines the extent of the injury (see pages 92, 94, 95).

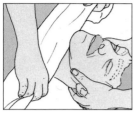

3 Place the collar gently on the casualty's neck, and bend it to wrap it around the sides of the neck, without pressing on the neck.

● Follow steps 1-4 for back injury, pages 94-95,

❶ Fold a newspaper or similar.

❷ Place this in a sling.

❸ Wrap it around the neck.

❹ Bring the ends forwards.

❺ Tie the ends to secure the collar.

❻ Monitor and reassure the casualty.

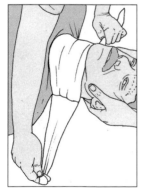

4 Pull the loose ends farther around the neck so that they come to the front. Keep a constant check on the casualty's breathing, pulse, and condition.

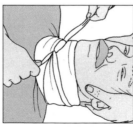

5 Tie the ends at the front, to give firm support to the neck, without undue pressure. Reassure the casualty that medical help will soon be available.

6 Keep the casualty warm and comfortable. If movement is essential, keep the neck and back in the same relative positions (see page 95).

CRUSH INJURIES

The main priority is to get emergency help — by shouting, waving, asking passers-by, using a phone, or any other means.

❶ Test the weight of an object before you try to move it.

❷ Get help by any means, then stay with the casualty.

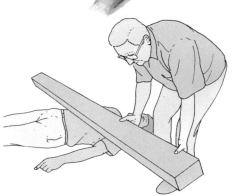

1 Test the weight of the fallen object, before you try to move it. You may be able to improvize a lever from a pole, girder, or similar, raising the object enough for the casualty to slide free. Otherwise, leave it in position.

2 Beware injuring yourself in trying to move the object. Try to attract attention and get help by any method, such as shouting, waving, throwing, or splashing. Stay with and reassure the casualty if possible.

BROKEN RIBS

A broken rib may show only as a
bruise under the skin. Beware of a
punctured lung (see page 78).

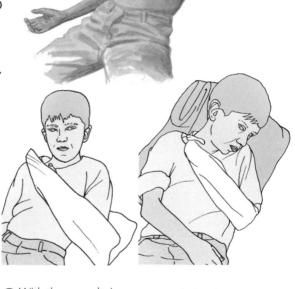

1 Place a pad over the
site, held by the
casualty's arm.

2 Apply a strap
or bandage
to hold the
pad and arm.

3 Get medical
attention.

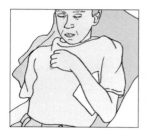

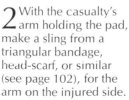

1 Lean the casualty to
the injured side, to
ease breathing. Call for
medical aid, or arrange
transport to hospital.
Place a large pad over
the injured site.

2 With the casualty's
arm holding the pad,
make a sling from a
triangular bandage,
head-scarf, or similar
(see page 102), for the
arm on the injured side.

3 Finish the sling to
support the arm and
hold the pad in place.
Check breathing (see
page 28). Call for
medical help or arrange
transport to hospital.

BROKEN NOSE OR CHEEKBONE

Broken nose
The nose has no true bone, but its stiff inner supporting plates of cartilage may be bent or cracked. Hospital attention is needed.

Broken cheekbone
The cheek (zygomatic) bone runs under the eye. If broken, it may cause swelling that affects the airway, so hospital attention is needed.

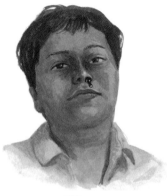

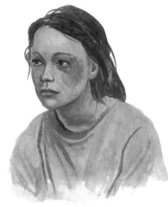

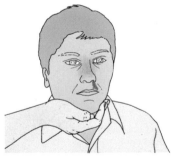

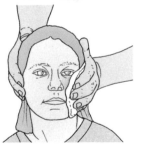

Give the casualty tissues or similar to wipe away blood and fluids. Do not try to unblock the nostrils. Call for emergency help, or arrange for transport to hospital. Support the jaw, which may also be damaged, with a neck collar (see opposite).

Apply a cold, moist, non-fluffy compress, such as a towel soaked in cold water, to the site. Reassure the casualty and call for emergency medical aid, or arrange for transport to hospital. Refresh the compress to keep it cold while you are waiting.

BROKEN JAW

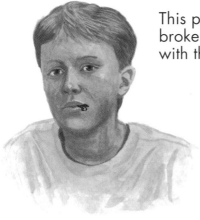

This painful injury may also involve broken teeth, which should be taken with the casualty to hospital.

❶ Assess the injury and collect any teeth (see page 75).

❷ Apply a neck collar (see page 96) and get to hospital.

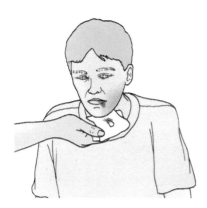

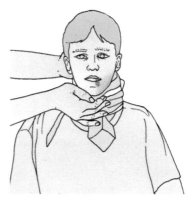

1 Wipe around the mouth and ensure that the casualty can breathe easily. Collect any broken or detached teeth and put them in a clean, damp cloth, to take to hospital. Arrange for medical help or transport to hospital.

2 Apply a support collar around the neck (see page 96) to stabilize and support the jaw. Reassure the casualty while waiting for medical aid, or take to hospital. The casualty should avoid speaking and any head or neck movements.

BROKEN COLLAR BONE

This injury can be caused by falling on the shoulder or outstretched arm.

Collar bone

1 Place arm across chest.

2 Find a triangular bandage.

3 Fold bandage under arm.

4 Tie ends on other shoulder.

5 Twist and tuck in point.

6 Adjust to support the arm.

7 Add a securing bandage around the chest.

8 Await medical help or go to hospital.

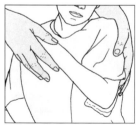

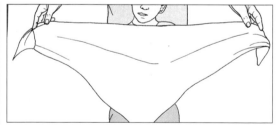

1 The collar bone in the upper front of the chest supports the shoulder. Take the strain from it by immobilizing the arm in a sling. Arrange medical help.

2 Use a triangular bandage or a folded head-scarf, towel, or similar. For a small casualty, fold it in half. Hold it centred on the body, longest edge

uppermost and horizontal. The casualty will probably hold the arm in the least painful position (see page 106), with the forearm angled across the chest.

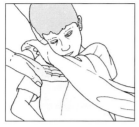 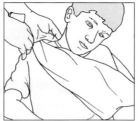 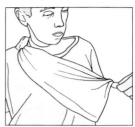

3 Fold the middle of the bandage around the arm on the injured side, so that one long point goes across the chest to the opposite shoulder.

4 Bring the other long point around the back of the neck. Tie the points together in a knot that sits in the hollow of the casualty's uninjured shoulder.

5 Twist the short point of the bandage to tighten it at the elbow and then tuck it in, so that the elbow cannot slip out.

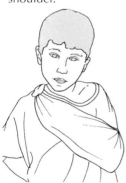 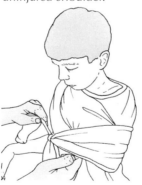 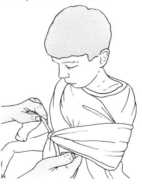

6 The completed sling should support and steady the arm, to relieve strain on the shoulder and collar bone, and immobilize the whole area.

7 Add a wide securing bandage, scarf, or similar around the upper arm on the injured side, and across the chest and upper back. Tie in place.

8 The casualty may now be able to walk. Wait for expert help to arrive or transport the casualty to hospital, avoiding sudden head or neck movements.

BROKEN ARM

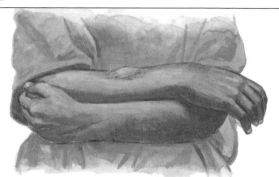

Call for medical aid as soon as possible. If this is delayed, or if the casualty will have to walk, consider applying a sling.

❶ Assess the extent of the injury. Support the injured arm. Arrange for medical attention.

❷ Place a pad over the area and wound (if it is an open fracture, see page 114).

❸ Secure the pad in place, but not too tightly.

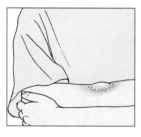

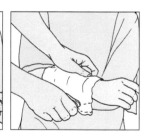

1 Assess the extent of the injury. Ask the casualty to support the injured arm with the uninjured one. Get medical help or arrange transport to hospital.

2 Place a large sterile or clean pad over the wounded area for protection. Keep the casualty calm, still, and quiet, and give reassurance.

3 Secure the pad at its ends with a strap, tape, bandage, or similar. Do not secure it too tightly and avoid direct pressure on the injury site.

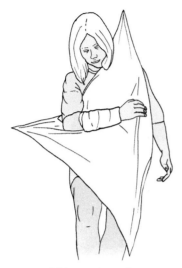

4 Use a triangular bandage or a folded head-scarf, towel, or similar. Slide it behind the injured arm, long edge vertical and short point near the elbow.

4 Prepare a triangular bandage or similar as a sling.

5 Complete the sling to support the injured arm.

6 Wait for medical help and reassure the casualty, or transport the casualty carefully to hospital.

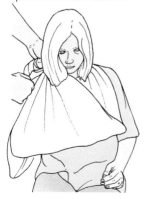

5 Fold the lower part of the bandage up over the arm and the upper part behind the neck. Tie the ends at the side with the knot in the hollow of the shoulder, to support the arm.

6 Twist the short point to tighten it against the elbow. Tuck it beside the elbow. Monitor the casualty's condition. Add a securing bandage (see page 103) if the casualty is to be moved.

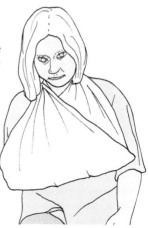

INJURED ELBOW

This treatment is for a broken arm bone near the elbow, or a dislocated or badly strained elbow joint. The aim is to immobilize the arm while waiting for expert help.

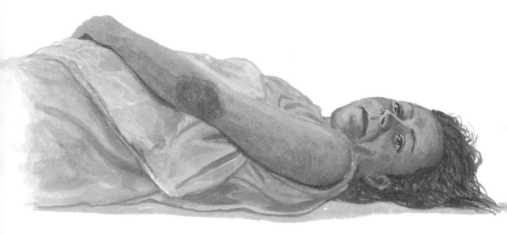

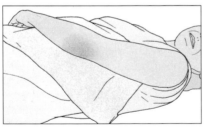

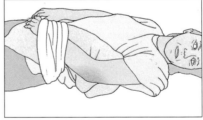

1 The casualty usually holds an injured part in the least painful position, so try to stabilize it in this posture (a general first aid principle known as "bind as you find"). Examine the area and place pads between the arm and body.

2 Get emergency medical help at the first opportunity, since it is unlikely the casualty will be mobile. Strap the injured area loosely to the body with the pads between, using a broad bandage, scarf, or similar item. Tie or knot on the uninjured side.

1 Assess the extent of the injury. Call for emergency medical help. Place pads between the elbow and the side of the body, adopting "bind as you find".

2 Bandage or strap the lower arm loosely to the side of the body.

3 Add a firmer strap or bandage above the injured area, around the upper arm, and strap to the body.

4 Repeat step 3 just below the elbow. Reassure the casualty, wait for help.

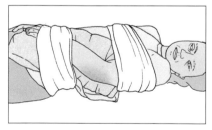

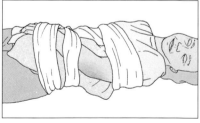

3 Put another broad strap or bandage across the upper arm and tie this more firmly. Reassure the casualty that help is on its way. Regularly check the pulse in the wrist of the injured arm, and pass this information to the medical staff.

4 Add a third broad bandage or strap just below the injury, and strap firmly to the body. Make the casualty as warm and comfortable as possible, with a head cushion, but try not to change his or her overall posture. Await expert help.

INJURED WRIST

In the wrist, as in several body parts, it is difficult to distinguish a severe sprain from a dislocation or a break (see pages 92, 152). First aid treatment is the same.

1 Remove watch or bracelet. Support the wrist.

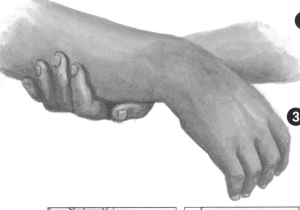

2 Immobilize with an improvized splint.

3 Support the arm in a sling. Get the casualty to hospital.

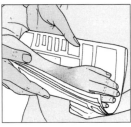 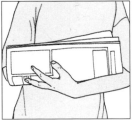 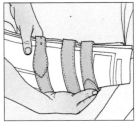

1 An injured wrist swells rapidly, with pain and loss of movement, so take off a watch, bracelet or ring. Use folded paper or similar as a splint.

2 Ask the casualty to hold the splint with the uninjured hand, so that you can strap it with a belt, bandage, or similar item, to immobilize the area.

3 After strapping, if the casualty has to walk some distance, put the arm in a sling (see page 105). Get medical help or arrange for transport to hospital.

INJURED FINGER

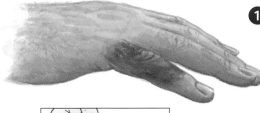

1 Remove rings if they are loose. Support the injured finger with an uninjured one.

2 Tie or strap the fingers together.

3 Make sure the ties are not too tight.

4 Get hospital attention.

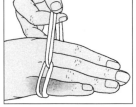

1 Remove rings if they are loose. Obtain a shoelace, thin rope, sticking tape, string, or similar for strapping.

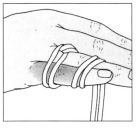

2 Use the adjacent uninjured finger as a splint. Tie or tape the fingers loosely together, with knots on the uninjured side. (See also page 148.)

3 Ensure the ties or tapes are firm but not tight, otherwise they may cut off the blood circulation, especially if the finger swells from its injury.

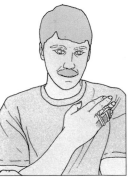

4 The casualty can hold the hand on the chest in a raised position, or support it in a sling (see page 105). Obtain medical help or take to hospital.

INJURED ANKLE

First aid is the same for a sprain or break (see page 92).

1 Assess the symptoms, improvize a splint.

2 Apply the splint to support the ankle.

3 Tie the splint to immobilize the area.

4 Get hospital attention.

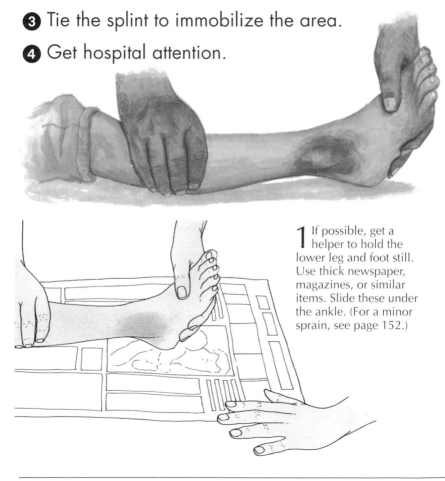

1 If possible, get a helper to hold the lower leg and foot still. Use thick newspaper, magazines, or similar items. Slide these under the ankle. (For a minor sprain, see page 152.)

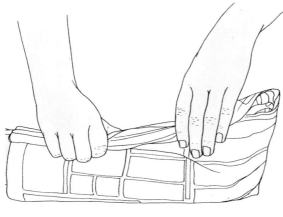

2 Fold the paper over the top of the foot, ankle, and shin, to support and immobilize the ankle joint. Try to keep the natural L shape of the joint.

3 Keep the splinting in place with belts, string, sticking tape, bandages, or similar items. Arrange for medical help or for transport to hospital.

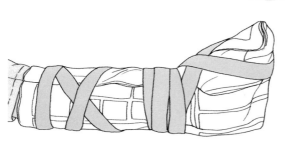

4 Once the ankle is fully splinted, the casualty may be able hobble on the uninjured foot, with help and support from others. Await medical assistance or take the casualty to hospital.

INJURED KNEE

The knee is the body's largest single joint, and a bad sprain, dislocation, or break is extremely painful. Get emergency medical attention.

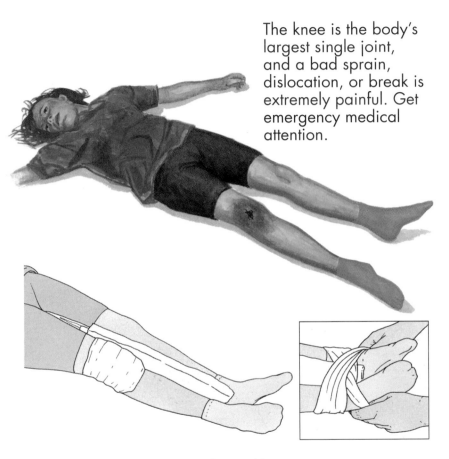

1 Deal with bleeding from wounds with large pads or similar dressings, but do not put direct pressure on the area. Get medical help as soon as you can. Put long padding between the legs, from the ankle to well above the knee. Use pillows, cushions, folded coats, or similar. Place the uninjured leg alongside.

2 Strap the ankles together with a bandage, belt, scarf, or similar item. Reassure the casualty that medical help is on its way.

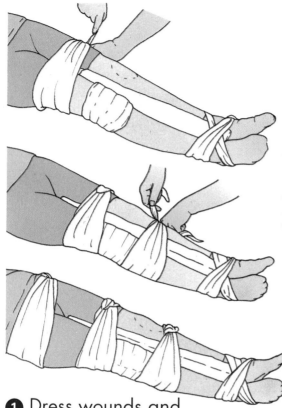

3 Strap the thighs together with a broad bandage, scarf, or similar. Put the strapping under the small of the back, and then ease it down.

4 Add further strapping around the shin and calf, below the injured area. Monitor the casualty's condition and beware of the signs of shock (see page 56).

5 Add another strap or bandage around the hip area. Keep the casualty warm (but not overheated), calm, and lying still while you wait for medical help. (For minor sprains, see page 152.)

1 Dress wounds and put long padding between the legs. Get medical help.

2 Strap the ankles, using the uninjured leg as a splint.

3 4 Add more straps.

5 Keep the casualty warm and calm, and await help.

OPEN (COMPOUND) FRACTURE

In an open (or compound) fracture, the skin is broken and the bones and tissues are exposed to the air, dirt, and other contamination. This brings the risk of infection and allows blood loss. Priorities are to cover the wound with sterile or clean dressings, to reduce the chance of contamination, and to send for emergency medical help. Keep the casualty still and reassured.

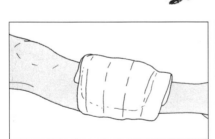

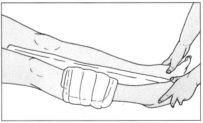

1 Cover the wounded area with large pads, either proper sterile dressings, or towels or similar items which are as clean as possible. Tape or bandage these loosely in place, avoiding direct pressure. Call for emergency help as soon as possible.

2 Keep any fragments or splinters of bone in a clean cloth, for grafting. Place padding between the legs, such as a pillow, cushions, a rolled-up blanket or coat, or similar. Bring the uninjured leg alongside the injured one, to act as a splint.

1 Cover the wound with sterile or clean pads. Fix these loosely. Avoid direct pressure to stop bleeding (for indirect pressure, see page 84). Get emergency medical help.

2 Pad between the legs, and use the uninjured leg as a splint.

3 Strap the legs, avoiding the injured area.

4 Monitor and reassure the casualty while waiting for assistance.

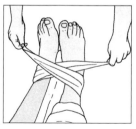 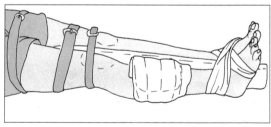

3 Strap the ankles using a bandage, belt, scarf, or similar. Pass it under the natural hollow above the heel, to avoid moving the leg. Add more straps.

4 Put strapping above the injured area. Place knots on the uninjured side, and do not strap directly over the wounded area. Keep the casualty warm, calm, and still, and reassure him or her that medical help is coming. Monitor the breathing and pulse, and watch for signs of shock (see page 56).

BROKEN THIGH OR HIP

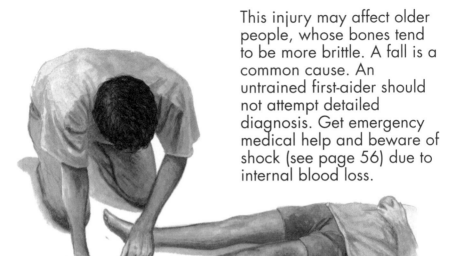

This injury may affect older people, whose bones tend to be more brittle. A fall is a common cause. An untrained first-aider should not attempt detailed diagnosis. Get emergency medical help and beware of shock (see page 56) due to internal blood loss.

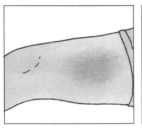 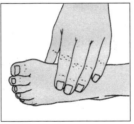 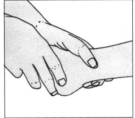

1 The injured area may swell rapidly and develop redness and bruising. The casualty will probably be in great pain. Call for emergency medical aid.

2 Remove footwear and feel for a pulse on the top of the foot. If this is absent, the main arteries carrying blood into the leg may be compressed or kinked.

3 If there is no foot pulse, pull gently on the foot to straighten the injured leg (in-line traction). Keep up the tension while a helper splints and straps the leg.

1 Assess the extent of the injury. Call for emergency medical help as soon as possible.

2 Check the blood supply to the lower leg.

3 If the pulse is absent, stretch the leg gently (in-line traction) with the aim of straightening the whole leg.

4 Place padding around the injured side.

5 Add a rigid splint to give extra support.

continued ▶

4 Make a U-shaped pad using a rolled-up blanket, coat, or similar. Place this around the injured leg. Or use separate pads to give the same effect.

5 Add a more rigid splint such as a walking stick, umbrella, strip of wood, or similar. Place this alongside the padding of the injured leg. Monitor the casualty's condition.

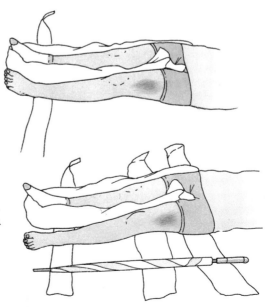

Broken thigh or hip continued

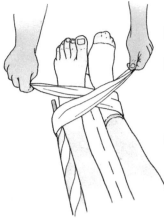

6 Strap the two ankles.

7 Add more straps, but not over the injury, so the uninjured leg gives support.

8 Keep the casualty still, warm, quiet, and reassured. Monitor his or her condition while waiting for assistance.

6 Strap the ankles together with a bandage, scarf, belt, rolled towel, or similar item. Keep the casualty warm, still, and reassured.

7 Add further strapping along the leg, but not directly over the injured area. For a suspected broken hip, splint and strap up to the high waistline.

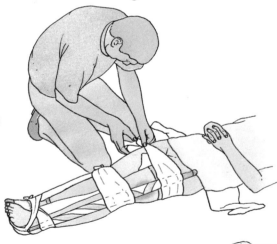

8 Check the casualty's condition while waiting for emergency assistance. Watch for signs of shock (see page 56) and continue to monitor the foot pulse.

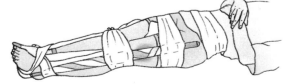

DEALING WITH BURNS

When there are burns and other fire injuries involved, tell the emergency medical services, so that they can bring suitable equipment and dressings.

First aid involves mainly cooling and protecting. If the burned skin is not broken, cool the area as rapidly as possible. For example, hold it under cold running water from a tap for about 10 minutes. This draws the heat from the tissues and reduces subsequent damage. After cooling, dress the area with a loose, dampened, preferably sterile pad. Do not bandage tightly.

If the skin is broken or burned away, cover the area with a clean pad for protection and to reduce the risk of infection, and get emergency help.

There are guides to assessing the depth of tissues affected by a burn (its degree), and the percentage of the body burned. But it is safest to get medical advice and attention, unless the burn is very small and does not break the skin. (For smoke inhalation, see page 52.)

WHAT TO DO IN CASE OF FIRE

❶ Get people clear as rapidly as possible. Do not be tempted to gather belongings or delay in other ways.

❷ Set off any fire alarm. Call the fire brigade or other emergency services. Warn others nearby of the danger.

❸ Give first aid to anyone burned or otherwise harmed.

❹ If your escape route is cut off, go into a room farthest from the fire, and close all connecting doors and windows.

❺ Stop the fire spreading by closing doors and windows, so it cannot feed off oxygen in fresh air.

❻ For a small fire, use an extinguisher. Point it at the base of the flames. Or smother the flames with a fire blanket.

CLOTHING ON FIRE

Do not let the casualty run about — this fans the flames. Smother the flames with a large blanket, coat, rug, or similar item. Get emergency help.

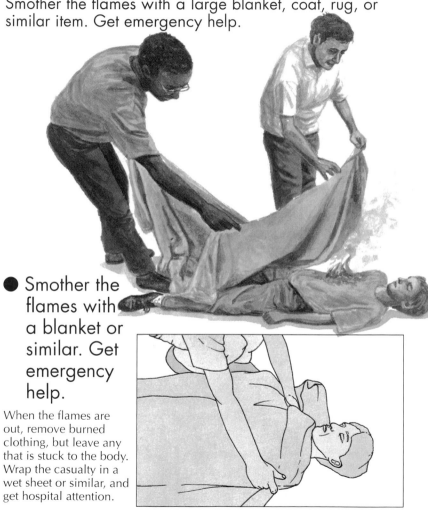

● Smother the flames with a blanket or similar. Get emergency help.

When the flames are out, remove burned clothing, but leave any that is stuck to the body. Wrap the casualty in a wet sheet or similar, and get hospital attention.

BLISTERS

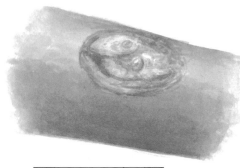

Blisters may form on a burned area or as a result of rubbing and friction. Cool and protect the area.

❶ Run cold water on the area (see page 120).

❷ Remove restrictive items in case of swelling.

❸ Wrap in a suitable dressing. Get medical attention.

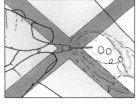

WARNING
Do <u>not</u> burst blisters

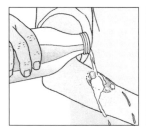

1 Run or pour cold water onto the area, from a tap, jug, river, or other source, for 10 minutes. Do not prick or burst the blister due to the risk of infection.

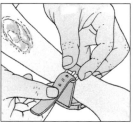

2 Remove watches, bracelets, rings, and other items that may cause problems if the area swells. Continue to cool the blister with cold water.

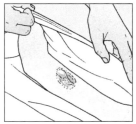

3 Cover the blister loosely with a non-stick dressing or a dampened, preferably sterile pad. Unless the blister is small, get the casualty to a doctor.

SCALDS (WET BURNS)

A scald is a burn caused by hot liquid. First aid is basically the same as for dry burns (see page 120).

1 Run cold water onto the area.

2 Remove restrictive items in case of swelling.

3 Wrap in a damp, clean pad. Get medical attention.

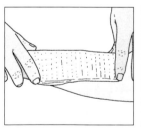

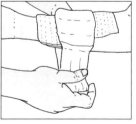

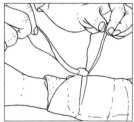

1 Cool the area with cold water for 10 minutes (see step 1, opposite). This also washes away the hot liquid. Cover with a clean, damp dressing.

2 Remove watches, bracelets, rings, and other items in case the area swells. Tape or bandage the dressing loosely in position. Do not apply pressure.

3 Tie the bandage loosely on the other side from the burned area. Unless the scalded area is very small, get the casualty to hospital or a medical centre.

MOUTH BURNS

These may be caused by very hot drinks or by steam from a kettle. Act fast since swelling may affect the breathing airway.

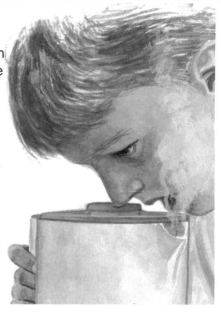

1 Get the casualty away from the heat, to a cooler place.

2 Call for emergency help. The casualty should lie in the stable side position (see page 40).

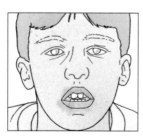

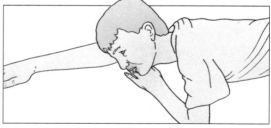

1 There may be burn or scald marks, redness, swelling around the lips and in the mouth, and perhaps in the nose. This can restrict breathing.

2 Get the casualty to a cooler place and ask him or her to lie in the stable side (recovery) position (see page 40). Call for emergency medical help. Reassure the casualty while you are waiting. The casualty may well be kept in hospital in case the swelling develops and blocks the breathing passages.

CHEMICALS IN THE EYE

If a chemical gets into the eye (except CS riot gas), flood the eye at once with water. Do not delay by trying to find a neutralizing substance.

❶ Flood the eye with clean water for as long as possible (1 hour).

❷ Apply pads, light bandage.

❸ Get the casualty to a hospital or medical centre.

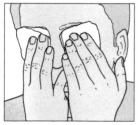

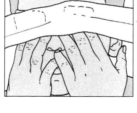

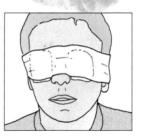

1 Flood the eye for up to an hour, or until skilled help arrives. The casualty should blink a lot. Ensure water drains away from the other eye. Apply damp pads.

2 Cover both eyes to reduce coordinated eye movements (see page 73). Explain this to the casualty. Secure the pads in place with a light bandage or tape.

3 Obtain emergency help or arrange for urgent transport to a hospital or medical centre. Inform the staff about the type of chemical involved.

ELECTROCUTION

Electricity may still be passing through the casualty (see page 14). Switch it off at the source, or knock the wire or appliance from the body with a wooden or plastic object (chair, broom).

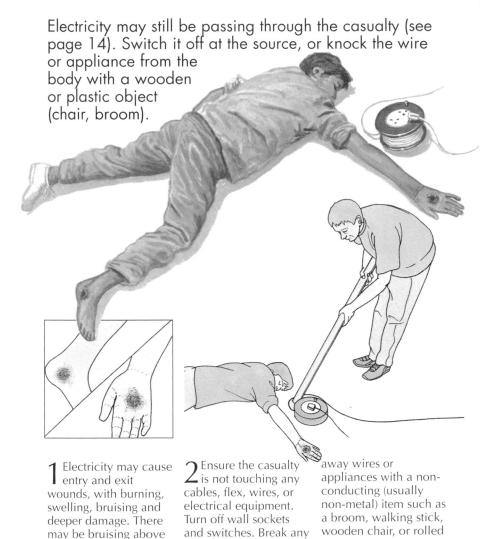

1 Electricity may cause entry and exit wounds, with burning, swelling, bruising and deeper damage. There may be bruising above the exit wound.

2 Ensure the casualty is not touching any cables, flex, wires, or electrical equipment. Turn off wall sockets and switches. Break any contact by knocking away wires or appliances with a non-conducting (usually non-metal) item such as a broom, walking stick, wooden chair, or rolled newspaper.

ELECTRICAL BURNS

❶ Electricity can cause deep burns, especially where it enters and leaves the body. It may also affect the heart and breathing, and send the body muscles into spasm.

❷ Break any contact between the electricity supply and the casualty, or you may also receive a shock and burns when you touch the casualty.

❸ Check the casualty and resuscitate if necessary. Put him or her in the stable side position. Get emergency medical help. There is no immediate treatment for the burns.

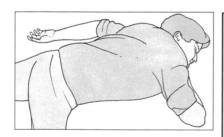

3 If the casualty is unconscious, check breathing and pulse, and resuscitate if necessary (see page 28). Place him or her in the stable side position (see page 40). Call for emergency medical help. Stay with and monitor the casualty.

ELECTRICITY AND SAFETY
● Ensure all electrical equipment and appliances are regularly checked. If in doubt, consult a qualified electrician.
● Replace frayed or kinked flex and cracked or broken plugs.
● Always unplug an appliance before adjusting or doing any work on it.
● Use circuit breakers and similar safety devices.
● Switch off at the consumer unit ("fuse board") before dealing with wall sockets and switches.

HEAT STROKE (HYPERTHERMIA)

In hot, humid conditions, the human body may not be able to cool itself sufficiently, especially if it is very active. It overheats and the person becomes ill and confused, and may collapse. (For heat exhaustion, see page 130).

Typically red, flushed, dry face

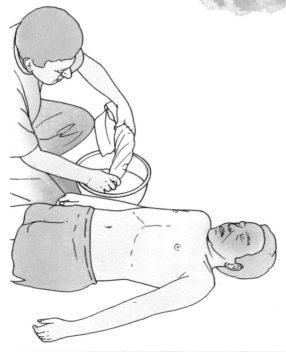

1 The priority is to cool the sufferer's body, whose temperature may exceed 40°C (104°F). Get the sufferer to a cooler, shady place and remove clothing. Find a sheet, towel, or similar covering, soak it in cold water and wring it out.

❶ Get the sufferer to a cooler, shady place.

❷ Cool the sufferer by various means, such as covering with a damp sheet and fanning.

❸ Monitor the sufferer's condition, and do not allow him or her to become chilled. Give plenty of fluids. Get medical advice.

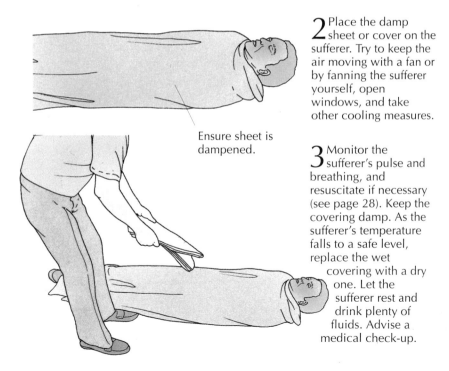

Ensure sheet is dampened.

2 Place the damp sheet or cover on the sufferer. Try to keep the air moving with a fan or by fanning the sufferer yourself, open windows, and take other cooling measures.

3 Monitor the sufferer's pulse and breathing, and resuscitate if necessary (see page 28). Keep the covering damp. As the sufferer's temperature falls to a safe level, replace the wet covering with a dry one. Let the sufferer rest and drink plenty of fluids. Advise a medical check-up.

HEAT EXHAUSTION

This condition involves loss of body fluids, salts, and minerals, as well as overheating. (For heat stroke, see page 128).

❶ Cool the sufferer and raise the legs.

❷ Give plenty of fluids and dilute salts.

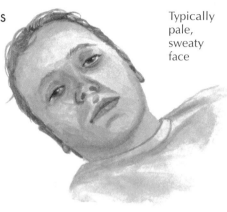

Typically pale, sweaty face

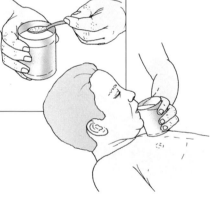

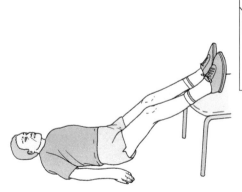

1 In heat exhaustion, the sufferer usually has a pale, clammy-looking face. Ask him or her to lie down in a cool, shaded place, with feet raised to encourage blood flow to the head and vital organs. Remove clothing and give reassurance.

2 Make a weak salt solution (1 spoon of table salt in 1 litre of clean water). Ask the casualty to sip this, up to 500 millilitres (250 for a child). He or she may drink plenty of plain, clean water. After recovery, advise a medical check-up.

HYPOTHERMIA

The body becomes too chilled and the sufferer may shiver, be confused, or collapse.

❶ Cover the sufferer.

❷ Re-warm the body gently, get medical attention.

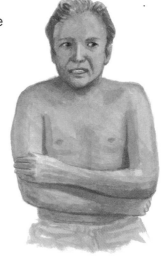

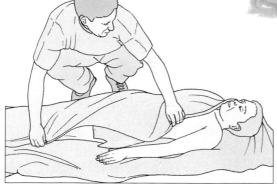

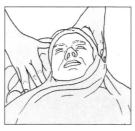

1 The sufferer should lie down, in a warm place if possible, and be wrapped in a blanket. Cover the head as well; much body warmth is lost from it. Use a silvery heat-retaining blanket, if available. Beware using hot-water bottles or a very nearby fire since the sufferer's skin may be numb, and burns might result.

2 Arrange for urgent medical attention. If the sufferer is conscious, he or she may sip a warm (not hot) drink. Do not give alcohol.

FROSTBITE

Intense cold freezes body tissues and damages their structures, nerves, and blood circulation, causing numbness and discolouration. The extremities are usually affected first, such as the toes, fingers, ears, and nose. As the parts thaw out, they become painful and swollen. Re-warm frostbitten parts gently and get medical attention.

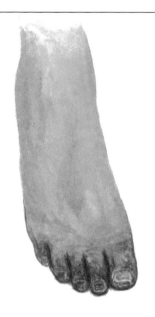

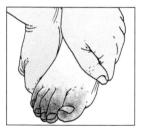 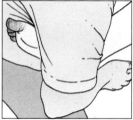 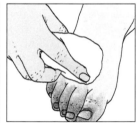

1 Transport the casualty to a warmer place if possible. Remove frozen garments and warm the affected parts by putting them next to the main body, under the armpit, between hands, or in a similar place, insulated from the cold. If you are in a remote area, continue this and send for emergency help.

2 Clean the area gently with warm water. Take great care since the thawed-out parts will be painful, and skin and flesh may come away.

❶ Re-warm the affected part so that it thaws slowly but thoroughly. Use heat from the main body, or immerse in a bowl of warm (not hot) water for a maximum of 3 minutes.

❷ Clean the area with warm water.

❸ Dry the area completely. Cover with a clean, loose pad.

❹ Add more pads and dressings, for protection, and to keep warmth in, and infection out.

❺ Arrange for the casualty to reach hospital.

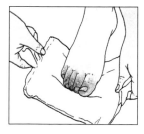

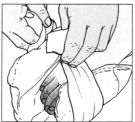

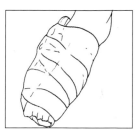

3 Make sure the area is thoroughly dry (even between the toes). Wrap the part in a sterile or clean loose pad or dressing, for warmth and protection.

4 Cover the area with more pads for further protection. Tape, bandage, or tie these loosely in place. Arrange for medical aid or transport to hospital.

5 Add the outer dressing, making sure it is not too tight. If the casualty must use the part, put minimal pressure on it. Get the casualty to hospital.

SUNBURN

Sunburn may be very painful and restricting, and ruin several days of valuable holiday time — yet it is nearly always avoidable. Follow the guidelines, and use a sunbarrier lotion or sunscreen cream appropriate for your skin type and previous exposure.

PREVENTING SUNBURN

● Consider if a suntan is so important, given the risks of sunburn, heat stroke, and various skin conditions, including possible growths and cancers.

● People with fair skin, freckles, and fair or reddish hair tend to burn more easily than those with dark skin and hair.

● On holiday, take it slowly at the start. Do not have more than 15-20 minutes of exposure to the sun on the first day. Increase this by 10-15 minutes daily.

● Follow the "Slip Slap Slop" routine. Slip on a T-shirt, slap on a sun hat, and slop on protective barrier lotion or screening cream.

● If you wish to sunbathe, do so when the sun's rays are least powerful, in the morning and evening. Avoid the intense sun of midday and early afternoon.

● The sun's UV rays can penetrate thin cloud and still cause burning.

Sunburn is basically the same as any other burn, with pain, redness, and swelling. Treat accordingly (see page 120). Watch the sufferer for signs of heat stroke (see page 128) or heat exhaustion (see page 130).

PART SIX

BITES, STINGS, POISONS, AND DRUGS

DOG BITES

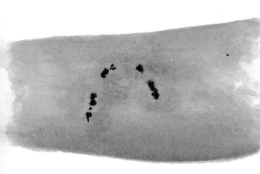

In some areas, the bite from a dog or similar animal carries the risk of rabies. If the skin is broken, get medical attention.

❶ Wash the wound well with water.

❷ Apply a clean dressing, attend hospital.

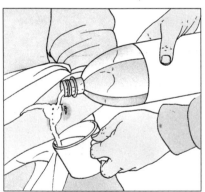

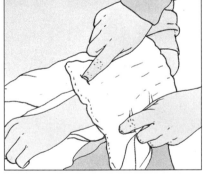

1 Ensure the dog or other animal is removed or under control, so that you and the casualty are not in further danger. Flood the wound and wash it well with clean water. Do not apply any commercial ointments or lotions.

2 Put a clean pad over the wound, and tape or bandage it in place. Call for medical help or take the casualty to a hospital or medical centre, for examination and possible injections against infection.

SNAKE BITES

Try to remember the snake's appearance, in case specific anti-venom is required. The casualty should keep still to avoid the poison spreading around the body.

❶ The wound usually shows as two small puncture marks. The casualty should avoid moving.

❷ Dress the wound, get to hospital.

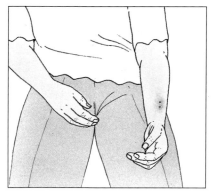

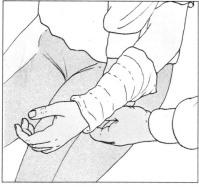

1 The casualty should sit down and rest, as still as possible. This reduces blood flow and delays the poison's spread. Arrange transport to hospital, call for medical help, or get telephone advice from a medical or poisons centre.

2 Apply a clean pad, and tape or bandage this loosely in place. Depending on the possible identity of the snake, follow expert advice. Await emergency help, or transport the casualty to a hospital or medical centre.

NETTLE RASH AND STINGS

This is usually a painful but temporary problem. Some people have a more severe allergic-type reaction (see opposite).

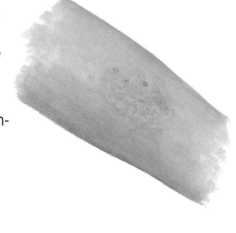

❶ Apply a suitable non-allergenic soothing lotion or cream.

❷ Some plants, like dock, can soothe.

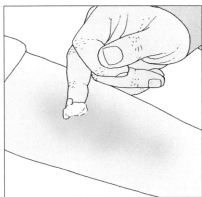

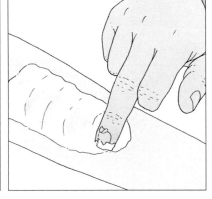

1 If a suitable non-allergenic anti-sting (anti-inflammatory) cream is available, rub this onto the site. There are also specific ointments and other preparations for nettle rash or sting. Or cool the redness and swelling with cold water.

2 Some wild plants, such as dock, help to soothe nettle stings. Rub the leaf gently onto the spots and raised lumps at the sting site. If the casualty has a severe reaction, see step 2 opposite.

BEE AND WASP STINGS

A bee leaves its sting in the skin; a wasp does not. Beware the severe reaction termed anaphylactic shock.

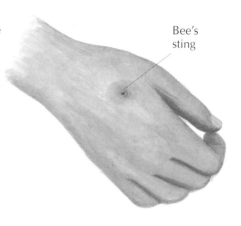

Bee's sting

❶ If the sting is visible, remove it with tweezers.

❷ Apply a cold pad, or anti-histamine or proprietary cream.

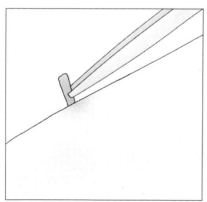

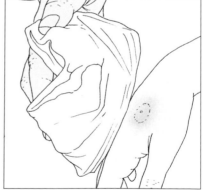

1 If you can see the small, dark sting, grasp its sharp tip and remove it with tweezers. Do not grab the bulging poison sac or this will inject more poison. Put a cold compress on the area, or apply anti-histamine or proprietary sting cream.

2 Rub the cream into the area. Severe allergic (anaphylactic) reaction may cause nausea, breathlessness, widespread swelling and possible collapse. Call for emergency help. Beware shock and resuscitate as necessary (see pages 28, 56).

JELLYFISH STINGS

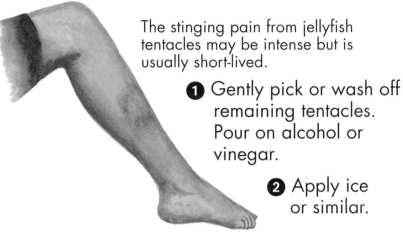

The stinging pain from jellyfish tentacles may be intense but is usually short-lived.

❶ Gently pick or wash off remaining tentacles. Pour on alcohol or vinegar.

❷ Apply ice or similar.

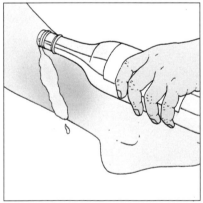

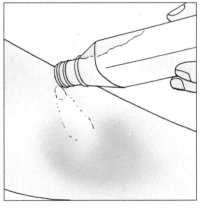

1 If you see any tentacles, gently pick them off with tweezers or clean fingernails. Wash with water. Pour on vinegar or alcohol, to help counteract the irritant chemicals in the sting. Keep the casualty still and quiet.

2 Cool the sting site with ice packs, chilled water or similar. If you see signs of severe reaction (anaphylactic shock, see page 139), get emergency help. If the pain does not subside in 1-2 hours, obtain medical advice.

SEA URCHIN STINGS

The tips of sea urchin spines may be so fine, they are almost invisible. The sting can be very painful, but usually fades. If pain persists or the site swells after several hours, get medical attention.

❶ Remove the spine if possible.

❷ Wash the part in hot water.

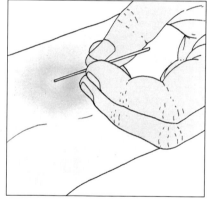

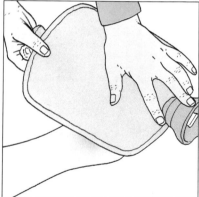

1 If you can see the spine embedded in the skin, pull it out. If this is not possible, get medical attention as soon as possible, or the spine may work its way deeper into the flesh. Keep the casualty calm and still.

2 Wash the site with hot water, apply a hot water bottle, or immerse the part in hot water for up to 30 minutes. This should help to draw out the venom. Monitor the casualty for anaphylactic shock (see page 139).

SWALLOWED CHEMICALS

The stomach is protected against its own natural corrosive chemicals; do not induce vomiting.

❶ Wash out the mouth with water.

❷ Make the casualty rest, get emergency help.

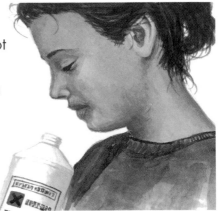

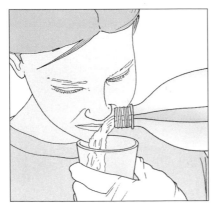

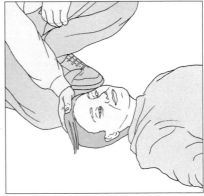

1 There may be redness in and around the mouth. Wash the mouth and lips with plenty of cold water, but do not let the casualty swallow this. Call for emergency help or get telephone advice from a hospital or poisons centre.

2 The casualty should lie down and rest. Monitor the pulse and breathing. Beware getting the chemical on yourself. Do not induce vomiting; the chemical will cause damage on the way out. Help medical staff to identify it.

POISONING BY PLANTS OR BERRIES

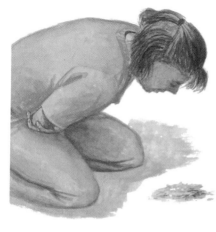

Nausea and vomiting are the body's natural way of ridding the digestive system of poisons.

❶ Encourage the casualty to vomit up the substances.

❷ Get medical aid, take a sample of the plant or vomit.

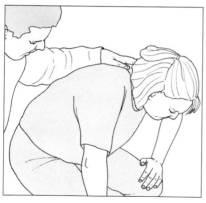

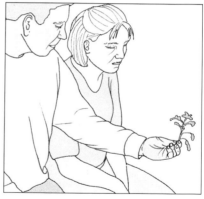

1 If the casualty feels sick, encourage him or her to vomit up the stomach contents and rid the body of the plant. If there is no nausea, but you are suspicious, arrange for transport to a hospital or medical centre for a check-up.

2 The casualty should not eat or drink. Take a sample of the plant, berries, mushrooms, or other substance with you, for identification by the medical staff. You may be able to get telephone advice from a poisons centre.

DRUG OVERDOSE

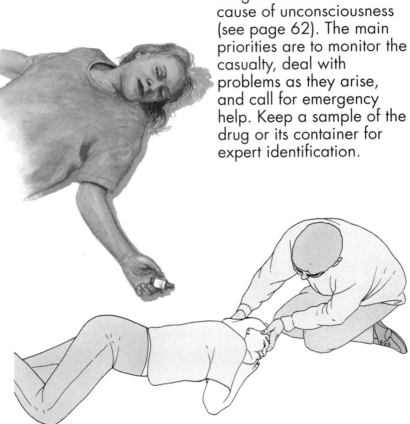

Drug overdose is one cause of unconsciousness (see page 62). The main priorities are to monitor the casualty, deal with problems as they arise, and call for emergency help. Keep a sample of the drug or its container for expert identification.

There may be clues to the nature of the overdose, such as a needle, powder, bottle, or container. Assess the casualty's condition and priorities (see page 12), monitor pulse and breathing, resuscitate if necessary (see page 28), and put the casualty in the stable side position (see page 40). Call for medical help or phone advice as soon as possible from a hospital, medical centre, or drugs unit. Keep any drugs, containers, equipment, and vomit for analysis and legal procedures.

SOLVENT ABUSE

The first aider should encourage the casualty to attend hospital and receive counselling and advice.

1 There may be signs such as a face rash.

2 Follow the advice for drug overdose (see opposite).

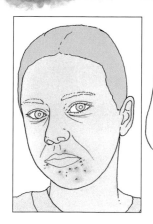

1 An habitual "glue-sniffer" develops spots and rash around the mouth from contact with the solvent substance. There may be plastic bags nearby.

2 If the casualty is unconscious, carry out an examination and follow main priorities (see page 12). Monitor the vital signs and resuscitate if necessary (see page 28), but beware breathing in the fumes yourself. Call for emergency help. If the casualty is conscious, encourage him or her to receive medical help.

DIABETIC CONDITIONS

In the condition called diabetes, the body does not produce one of its natural hormones (chemicals), called insulin. This hormone normally controls the level of blood sugar, which provides the body with energy. Lack of insulin means the blood sugar level is not adjusted properly. Diabetic people may eat a controlled diet, and take tablets and/or injections, to keep the level of blood sugar stable. Sometimes this treatment is disrupted, for example by illness, fatigue, or unfamiliar foods.

In hypoglycaemia, the blood sugar level becomes too low. The person may feel faint, dizzy, confused, and possibly appear drunk or aggressive. He or she has pale, sweaty skin, rapid pulse, shallow breathing, and tremors, and may collapse. Call for emergency help. Ask for advice from medical staff. Monitor the person (see page 28). If he or she is conscious, carefully give sweet or sugary drinks or foods.

CLUES AT THE SCENE
If you see these items at the scene of an accident, or associated with a casualty, he or she may be diabetic. Inform medical staff.

● Insulin syringe and case

● Blood and urine testers

● Medic Alert warning badge or bracelet

● Novo-pen insulin injector

● HypoStop fast-acting sugar gel (rub onto gums)

PART SEVEN

OTHER CONDITIONS

TRAPPED FINGERS

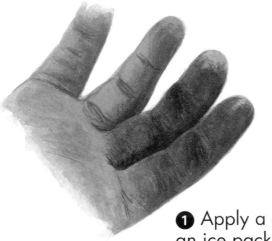

The skin and tissues of the fingers are very sensitive to touch and pain. Squashing them in a door or under a weight can be very uncomfortable! (For broken finger, see page 109.)

❶ Apply a cold compress or an ice pack to reduce swelling.

❷ Apply a dressing.

❸ Raise and support the hand.

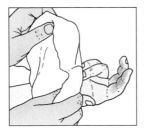

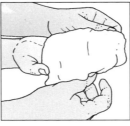

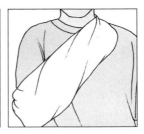

1 Remove rings or other restrictive items. Cool the fingers with a cold compress, crushed ice in a plastic bag, or a frozen food pack.

2 Cover the fingers with a pad, and tape or bandage this loosely in position. If the casualty has lost any movement or feeling, arrange for medical aid.

3 Support the hand in a raised (elevated) position using a sling (see page 102). If the swelling and pain persist after a few hours, seek medical advice.

MUSCLE CRAMPS

Cramp is uncontrolled spasm (contraction) of a muscle, making it tense and rigid, due to build-up of lactic acid.

❶ Massage and rub the muscle well.

❷ Stretch the muscle slightly.

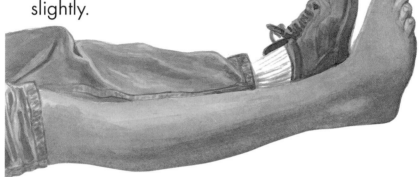

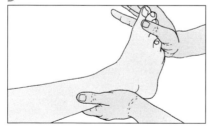

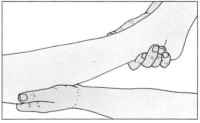

1 Cramp can occur in almost any muscle, often as a result of unaccustomed activity. It is common in the gastrocnemius muscle in the calf. The casualty should sit or lie down, as you rub and massage the muscle.

2 Stretch the muscle gently by pulling against its contraction, in this case, bending the foot towards the shin. Massage and stretching increase blood flow to the muscle, to carry away and disperse the lactic acid.

SPLINTERS

Fragments of wood, metal, or other substances may become embedded in the skin. If swelling and pain persist, seek medical aid.

❶ Clean the area and remove the splinter.

❷ Squeeze to promote bleeding, dress the wound.

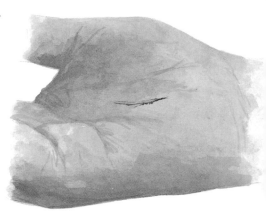

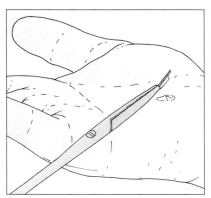

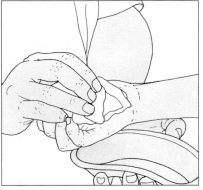

1 Wash the area clean with soap and warm water. Sterilize the tips of fine tweezers or a needle point in a flame. When cool, try to grasp and pull out the splinter, or lever it out from below. Ask the casualty to remain still, if possible!

2 Squeeze the area to encourage bleeding which should wash any remaining fragments from the wound. Clean the area again with soap and water, and apply a sticking plaster or dressing as for a wound (see page 77).

SUPERGLUE ACCIDENTS

Modern fast-acting cyano-acrylate "superglues" need very careful handling. They can bond skin, eyelids, lashes, nails, or other body tissues in seconds. Get the casualty to hospital urgently.

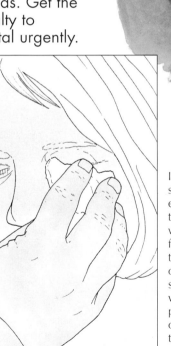

If superglue affects a delicate or sensitive part, such as sticking the eyelids together, do not try to prise them apart. Bathe the area with warm water, ensure there are no further drops of glue around, and then take the casualty to a hospital or medical centre. If the fingers get stuck, wash these with warm, soapy water and, gently and slowly, try to prise them apart. The surface flakes of skin may pull away and allow this to happen. If not, seek medical aid.

MINOR SPRAINS AND STRAINS

A variety of minor injuries go by these names. They are painful, but they do not normally affect the degree of movement or feeling (touch sensation). For more serious injuries, see Part Four (page 92).

1 Support the injured part.

2 Strap or tape the support or splint in place.

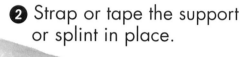

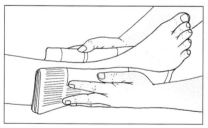

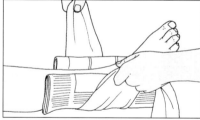

1 Almost any body part can be affected by a minor sprain or strain, but these problems are most common in the limbs. This example shows an ankle sprain (see also page 110), but the principles apply to all parts. Improvize a support.

2 The support or splint may be folded or rolled newspaper, thick pads, pieces of wood, or similar items. Check the injury is not too serious, with no open wound or obvious bone deformity. Begin to strap the support.

❸ Ensure that the support is not too tight, so that it can permit swelling.

❹ Finish securing the support or splint. Check the amount of swelling and bruising.

❺ If the problem persists, seek medical advice.

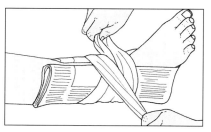

3 Use bandages, scarves, towels, belts, or similar items to strap the support. Put these above and below the injured area, but not directly over it. Leave the support or splint slightly loose, so that there is room for further swelling.

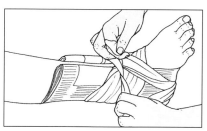

4 In this example, a triangular bandage has been strapped in figure-8 fashion to secure the support of a rolled-up newspaper. Check that bruising and swelling are not too severe, and that the casualty can move and feel the part.

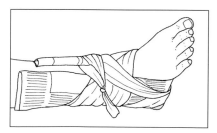

5 Keep weight and pressure off the injured part. If the pain persists or worsens after several hours, the problem may be a more serious dislocation or fracture. Take the casualty to a hospital or medical centre for a detailed examination.

EMERGENCY CHILDBIRTH

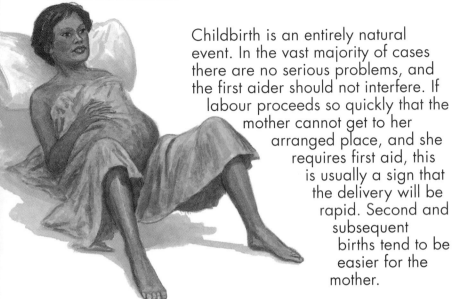

Childbirth is an entirely natural event. In the vast majority of cases there are no serious problems, and the first aider should not interfere. If labour proceeds so quickly that the mother cannot get to her arranged place, and she requires first aid, this is usually a sign that the delivery will be rapid. Second and subsequent births tend to be easier for the mother.

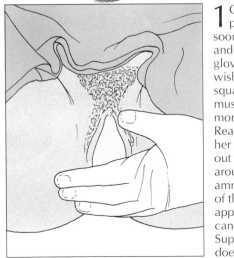

1 Get the mother to a safe, quiet place and call for medical help as soon as you can. Wash your hands and wear medical or clean rubber gloves, if possible. The mother may wish to lie back with knees raised, or squat. The contractions of the muscular womb (uterus) become more powerful and frequent. Reassure the mother and encourage her to pant between desires to push out the baby. The sac or membranes around the baby rupture, with loss of amniotic fluid, known as "breaking of the waters". The baby's head appears at the birth opening (vaginal canal). This is called crowning. Support the head so that the baby does not emerge too quickly.

❶ Get the mother to a quiet place. Encourage her to pant between the contractions of the womb with urges to push. Support the baby's head as it appears at the birth opening.

❷ Support the baby as it emerges. It should slide out without assistance.

❸ Wipe the baby's nose and mouth. *continued* ▶

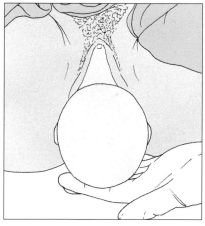 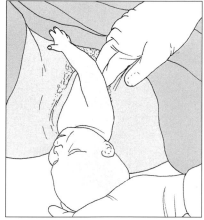

2 The head should emerge smoothly, turning as it appears. Support the baby as this stage of birth, called delivery, continues. If the umbilical cord is wrapped around the neck, you may have to try and untangle it, with great care.

3 Next comes the shoulder. The delivery speeds up and the rest of the baby usually emerges with another few contractions. Wipe any fluid or membranes from the baby's face, nose, and mouth. Hold it carefully since it is slippery.

Emergency childbirth continued

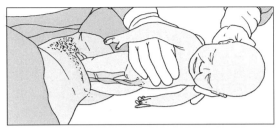

4 Lift the baby clear as the feet emerge. It should begin to breathe on its own. Keep it above the level of the placenta (afterbirth) which is still in the womb.

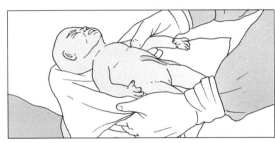

5 Pass the baby to the mother. This is a very important time for both. Do not cut the umbilical cord.

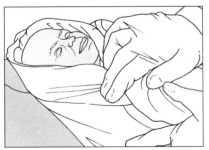

6 Wrap the baby in a clean towel, shawl, or similar item, to keep it warm. Cover the head, since much heat is lost from there, leaving the face clear. The baby may cry lustily or breathe quietly; either is quite natural.

7 The placenta (afterbirth) usually emerges about 10-15 minutes after the baby is born. Put it in a bowl or wrap it in a sheet, so that it can be examined later by medical staff. Do not cut the umbilical cord.

④ Lift the baby clear when it has fully emerged, keeping it above womb level.

⑤ Pass the baby to the mother, for important early mother-baby contact.

⑥ Wrap the baby to reduce heat loss, or it may soon become chilled, even in a warm room.

⑦ Monitor the delivery of the placenta (afterbirth). Keep this and do not cut the cord.

⑧ If the baby fails to start breathing, flick the soles of its feet.

⑨ Or rub its back, or try artificial ventilation.

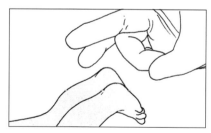 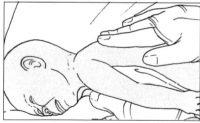

8 If the baby does not start to breathe properly as soon as it is is born, flick the soles of its feet with your fingers. This usually stimulates breathing. Fluids and mucus drain away naturally if the baby is face- and chest-down.

9 Rubbing the baby's back may also stimulate breathing. If breathing does not begin after a minute or two, try mouth-to-mouth-and-nose ventilation (see page 38). Stay with the mother and baby until help arrives.

INDEX